e-Health Care in Dentistry and Oral Medicine

Nicolas Giraudeau
Editor

e-Health Care in Dentistry and Oral Medicine

A Clinician's Guide

Springer

Editor
Nicolas Giraudeau
Public health, LBN EA 4203, Odontology,
University of Montpellier
Montpellier, France

ISBN 978-3-319-69449-8   ISBN 978-3-319-69450-4 (eBook)
https://doi.org/10.1007/978-3-319-69450-4

Library of Congress Control Number: 2017964626

Printed on acid-free paper

This Springer imprint is published by Springer Nature
The registered company is Springer International Publishing AG
The registered company address is: Gewerbestrasse 11, 6330 Cham, Switzerland

Contents

Part I

General Aspects of e-Oral Health

Definition of Teledentistry

1

Rodrigo Mariño and Aghareed Ghanim

Abstract

The concept of teledentistry proposes the application of a variety of information and communications technologies (ICT) to facilitate oral health care for geographically distant patients and/or practitioners. This chapter presents an overview of the uses of information and communication technologies in oral health. The first part defines teledentistry, addresses general concepts and provides an overview of teledentistry and its common uses in oral health. The final section describes some of the general health implications of teledentistry, explaining the role played by health professionals in promoting the uses of ICT in oral health and stimulating the need for further interdisciplinary research and education in teledentistry. The chapter aims to describe the foundation for teledentistry and underline its merits for the delivery of oral health care. The chapter also discusses the opportunities and benefits associated with the adoption of teledentistry solutions as well as its utilisation and impact on the oral health system and the population.

Keywords

ICT • Telehealth • Tele(oral)health • Teledentistry • e-health • e-(oral)health

1.1 Introduction

The use of communication technology to improve access to and quality of health care and to decrease inequalities in health has a long history. There has always been a connection between medicine/health and communication tools. For example, the use of a torch system to relay messages by the ancient Greeks [1], the use of sounds

R. Mariño (✉) • A. Ghanim
Melbourne Dental School, The University of Melbourne, Melbourne, 3010 Victoria, Australia
e-mail: r.marino@unimelb.edu.au

N. Giraudeau (ed.), *e-Health Care in Dentistry and Oral Medicine*,
https://doi.org/10.1007/978-3-319-69450-4_1

(drums, bells), the use of quipus (or talking knots, a complicated systems of recording and administration based on the use of strings) by the Incas, and smoke signals were all early attempts to exchange or communicate health information, news about major catastrophes or significant health events like the bubonic plague in Europe [2, 3]. Despite this, these are not considered examples of telemedicine [4].

According to Vladzymyrskyy and coresearchers, there is a strong connection between telemedicine and electrical and electronic communication tools [4]. Telemedicine started as soon as these technologies (telegraph, telephone and radio) were invented. Thus, it was not until the 1850s that technological advances for the transmission of information by telegraph, telephone and radio allowed for the expansion of telecommunication and informatics. From this perspective, the history of telemedicine, and probably the term itself, can be traced to the mid-nineteenth century. The telegraph was used during the American Civil War and in Central Australia in 1874, in which records show how the telegraph played an important telemedicine role in enabling care for wounded people [5]. Later, in the early twentieth century (1905), there was a transmission of an electrocardiogram (ECG) [6].

The prefix "tele" is derived from a Greek term which means "at a distance"; hence, more simply, telemedicine means "healing at a distance". The term was first used in 1927 in a newspaper article [4]. A few years earlier, in 1924, Hugo Gernsback described "teledactyl" [7], an early vision of telemedicine, where a doctor could use radio signals to generate a video image of the patient and remotely operate a robotic hand to examine the patient. In his vision, the doctor of the future could "feel at a distance". Back then it sounded like science fiction, but 90 years later it is a reality. Radiology images started being sent in the 1940s via telephone lines [7]. Nonetheless, it was not until the 1960s and 1970s when modern telecommunication technologies started expanding and being ubiquitous in our world that the term telemedicine started being used as largely military and space applications and the health care began demonstrating how information and communications technology (ICT) could provide new solutions in areas of shortage of specialists or lack of proper health care. Terms such as teleconsultation and telediagnosis start appearing in the 1970s. More recently, with the exponential growth of sensors and social applications, cloud, big data, etc. and the increasing familiarity of patients to these technologies, a demand has been created for anytime anywhere access to information and health care [8].

This chapter presents an overview of the uses of information and communication technologies in oral health. It is organised into three main sections; the first section will look at a definition of telemedicine and explore differences between e-health, telehealth and telemedicine and will present major areas of telehealth applications. The second section will expand on the definitions of telemedicine and teledentistry and will present the most common uses of teledentistry in oral health. The final section will describe some general health implications of teledentistry, explaining the role played by health professionals in promoting the uses of ICT in oral health and stimulating the need for further interdisciplinary research and education in teledentistry.

1.2 Telehealth and Telemedicine Defined

Just as the uses of ICT have developed over the years, the terms to describe health-care services at a distance, such as "telehealth", "e-health" and "telemedicine", have also evolved. Within this evolution, Standards Australia defines e-health, which is generally accepted as composed of two elements: (1) *health informatics*, which relates to the collection, analysis and movement of health information and data to support health care, and (2) *telehealth*, which relates to direct (e.g. videoconferencing) or indirect (e.g. website) delivery of health information or health care to a recipient [9].

E-health has also been defined by the World Health Organization (WHO) as the "cost-effective and secure use of information and communication technologies in support of health and health-related fields, including health-care services, health surveillance, health literature and health education, knowledge and research" [10]. However, WHO uses "telehealth" and "e-health" as umbrella terms "to encompass the rapidly evolving discipline of using computing, networking and communications - methodology and technology - to support the health related fields, such as medicine, nursing, pharmacy and dentistry" [11].

For the European community, e-health includes "products, systems and services that go beyond simply Internet-based applications. They include tools for both health authorities and professionals as well as personalised health systems for patients and citizens" [12]. Examples include electronic health records, telemedicine services, personal wearable and portable communicable systems, health portals and many other information and communication technology-based tools assisting prevention, diagnosis, treatment, health monitoring and lifestyle management [12].

Other components of e-health include the use of mobile devices, such as mobile phones, patient monitoring devices and other wireless devices, for medical and public health practices, and the use of rules, regulations, guidelines or definitions with technical specification to make the integrated management of health systems viable at all levels (standardisation and interoperability) [10].

Although some definitions suggest using telemedicine and telehealth as interchangeable terms, telemedicine is different from telehealth. Telehealth is broader in definition than telemedicine as it includes computer-assisted telecommunications to support management, surveillance, literature and access to medical and health knowledge [11]. Telemedicine is the use of telecommunications for any health-related activities carried out over distance by means of information communication technologies.

A definition of telemedicine is provided by the World Health Organization [11] as:

> The delivery of health care services, where distance is a critical factor, by all health care professionals using information and communication technologies for the exchange of valid information for diagnosis, treatment and prevention of disease and injuries, research and evaluation, and for the continuing education of health care providers, all in the interests of advancing the health of individuals and their communities.

This definition identifies four connected elements [11]:

- Its purpose is to provide clinical support.
- It is intended to overcome geographical barriers, connecting users who are not in the same physical location.
- It involves the use of various types of ICT.
- Its goal is to improve health outcomes.

Moreover, it establishes first and foremost that it is the delivery of health care through the use of ICT. It includes the potential to benefit health care by enhancing early diagnosis, facilitating timely treatment of oral diseases, reducing isolation of practitioners through communication with peers and specialists and improving access to care. It also includes the support of long-distance and remote patient and professional health-related education, public health and health administration. Additionally, other definitions specify that telemedicine [10]:

- Reduces inequalities
- Reduces costs and brings economic benefits
- Improves the quality of care
- Achieves socio-sanitary objectives (reduction of waiting lists, teleconsultation)

1.2.1 Telemedicine: Applications and Mechanism of Delivery

Given the breadth of this definition, telemedicine has a wide number of beneficial applications across medical fields and is firmly embedded within the broader area of telehealth. Table 1.1 outlines the variety of telehealth technology applications available.

Table 1.1 Major areas of telehealth technology applications

Teleconsultation Telediagnosis Tele-treatment	The patient, with the local health professions, consults the specialist and obtains the line of treatment
Tele-education Tele-training	For continuing professional development (CPD) and training for oral health professionals Methods for sharing scientific knowledge, such as e-publication, open access, digital literacy and the use of social networks
Tele-monitoring	Regular monitoring of physical and/or biochemical parameters in chronically ill patients (dialysis and cardiorespiratory patients, etc.) for intensive care and/or emergency care
Tele-support	Support to remote health facilities located in isolated areas, remote places or in areas affected by natural disasters, armed conflict, etc.
Tele-administration	Electronic medical records or electronic health record and the use of communications technology for purely administrative work (e.g. scheduling and managing appointments)
Consumer medical and health information	Websites used for both clinical and educational purposes combine different applications ranging from merely informative (static) pages to completely interactive applications

Sources: Modified from [13–15]

There are primarily three basic techniques that are used for telemedicine, according to the time when information is transmitted: real-time consultation, store and forward and near real time. Each has its own value for particular subspecialties in specific situations [16].

Real-time consultation, also known as synchronous, collects information which is transmitted and displayed with no delay between parties at the sites. Videoconferencing is a common method of real-time communication. The system could utilize audio-visual tools so that the users at either site can see and interact with each other. Individuals can share work space on their computer desktops. It might also be "application sharing", where a piece of software can be run and controlled by both parties [13].

The store and forward technique, also known as "asynchronous" or "pre-recorded" consultation, utilizes less complicated equipment and can operate via the Internet. The health professional collects all the necessary information and stores it in a file. The file is forwarded via e-mail, or other means. The consultant retrieves the file and examines its contents. Recommendations are then provided to the dental professional in the same manner in return [17].

Both real-time and store and forward techniques require the same basic types of hardware, software, peripheral devices and telecommunication links with appropriate bandwidth. They involve a dental care professional digitising and electronically transmitting videos, drawings, diagrams, photographs and X-rays to the distant site [18]. The true real-time consultation allows for a detailed discussion by personal contact and clarification of points as they arise. The availability of a camera allows for capturing snapshots even when images for 3D objects such as models are required [13]. Because of its special functional characteristics, when compared to the store-forward technique, real-time operations required faster connections, the deployed equipment are usually more sophisticated and expensive and an extremely high speed network connection is required which is not usually available outside of major municipal areas unless a satellite is utilized [16]. In contrast, the store and forward technique is much less expensive yet provides vast benefits for a wide range of applications and is just as effective at presenting cases in a real-time setting. It can be achieved using ordinary telephone lines. For many clinicians, store and forward form is acceptable, since it can also be difficult to arrange convenient times for real-time contact [13].

The near-real-time solution is a variant of the real-time mode where data sent ranges from low-resolution, low-frame-rate images to something that looks like jittery television [16]. This mode is applicable where network connections are poorer, when communication costs are high or when real-time communication is important, but data quality is not a critical issue. For example, this was the solution used by Mariño and his collaborators for sites that could not accommodate 3 Mbits/s stream [19]. In those cases, a store and forward version was developed that enabled the Mpeg4 file to be stored on a central server for asynchronous download a few minutes after the actual exam.

1.3 Teledentistry Defined

Commonly, teledentistry has incorporated the prefix "tele" to common dental clinical applications. Terms have evolved to describe the application of telehealth to those particular dental specialties, such as "teleprosthodontics", "teleperiodontology" "teleorthodontics", "tele-oral surgery" and "telepaedodontics". As a consequence, several definitions and descriptions of teledentistry are found in the literature, each highlighting some aspect of teledentistry [20–28]. Nonetheless, the use of a telemedicine definition helps to identify the realm of teledentistry as a branch of telehealth. More specifically, as the use of ICTs to support oral health-care delivery, and for the organisation, management and distribution of health information in support of patient and professional health-related education, practice, public health, research, health-care administration, information gathering and synthesis and knowledge sharing [14, 15, 29].

As such, it represents an intersection of traditional methods with ICT to meet oral health's clinical, administrative, research and educational needs. It allows better accessibility to oral health-care information and services to high-risk populations living in underserved areas. It also empowers and upskills local community oral health-care providers in rural areas who are able to access advice from specialists in major metro teaching hospitals and practices [30].

As mentioned, the use of electronically based information technologies in oral health is not new. As early as 1950, dental educators pioneered the use of closed circuit television and its facility for image amplification through electronics [31]. Dental continuing education courses were first distributed by video telecommunications via satellite transmissions in the 1960s, and in return of the growth of reimbursement for health-care services by third-party payers, the American Dental Association in 1969 invented and developed a standardised dental disease coding system which introduced automation and computer processing of claims for reimbursement for dental treatment [31]. This system today enjoys universal use by practitioners, demographers, insurance companies and government agencies. Still, compared to medicine, teledentistry is a relatively new area of health using ICT. Teledentistry remains under-used as a means of diagnosis, consultation and referral in everyday dental practice ICT applications.

Probably the largest teledentistry undertaking in the world is currently being performed by the US military [27]. The teledentistry-military project began in 1994 to serve the troops and their dependents around the world by improving their oral health and offering continuing dental education [32]. This project primarily deployed a conventional telephone system, with two different communication modalities: real time and store and forward. The project concluded that teledentistry decreased overall cost, was expandable to remote and rural areas, offered better care for patients than a traditional referral process and provided more complete information for data analysis [31].

1.3.1 Reasons for Teledentistry

Teledentistry has the potential to benefit oral health care by enhancing early diagnosis, facilitating timely treatment of oral diseases, reducing isolation of practitioners through communication with peers and specialists and improving access to care. People living in rural or underserved areas are among the most in need of oral health care in their communities [33, 34]. In addition to the lack of oral health-care providers in these areas, barriers to the accessibility of quality dental care appear to be geographical distance and limited local resources [27, 33–35]. Many rural communities lack the clinical settings and finances that are required to attract specialised dental providers. Patients living in rural areas who are referred to dental care providers in more urban settings must travel to these areas which is usually expensive and time-consuming. Teledentistry can close this distance gap by allowing oral health-care providers in the rural areas to seek advice from specialists in the urban settings [33, 34]. This can be performed without the patient having to physically enter the specialty practice.

At the current level of development, most teledentistry programmes have focused on distance management and administration of remote facilities, learning and continuing education and consultation and referral services rather than direct patient care. A review of the literature showed that teledentistry applications are highly diverse in both study context and methods applied [30]. Areas of intervention in teledentistry indicated that the most common types of intervention evaluated were oral and maxillofacial surgery, oral medicine and pathology, orthodontics, preventive dental care (i.e. oral health-care maintenance and interventions) and dental education in different disciplines but mainly orthodontic [30]. More recently, other dental specialties have also incorporated teledentistry uses. Still, fewer studies were conducted on paedodontics, periodontics and prosthodontics, oral and maxillofacial trauma, endodontics and other dental fields [30].

Furthermore, if dentistry parallels medicine, the areas of oral medicine (mucosal lesions) and chronic facial pain will be areas in which teleconsultations will be incorporated. Specialists who can treat orofacial disorders such as oral mucosal diseases, temporomandibular joint dysfunction, orofacial pain and oral medicine are not affordable in rural areas. These disorders are usually chronic conditions that need recurring visits and intense patient care [36].

Patients of all ages, children/parents to geriatrics, have reported high levels of satisfaction with teledentistry [19, 37]. In addition, several studies have demonstrated acceptable levels of equivalence between teleconsultation and face-to-face consultation [19, 38]. However, oral medicine consultation studies have found that a face-to-face patient assessment is more precise in establishing an appropriate diagnosis for oral mucosal disease than transmitted descriptive patient data alone as it was preferred to have seen more oral mucosal pathologies information [39, 40]. Nonetheless, at the current state of development of teledentistry, there is no replacement for face-to-face oral health care. Oral health professionals cannot treat the majority of oral health problems with a simple prescription, except where there is obvious infection. Instead, the patient must be referred for care. As such the type of clinical application typically undertaken in teledentistry focuses on tele-education, tele-diagnostic, teleconsultation and tele-treatment as the only applications [30]. Some studies have also incorporated tele-support and tele-monitoring. They represent some of the broad range of teledentistry clinical and non-clinical applications. Other applications included the combination of tele-diagnostic and tele-treatment, teleconsultation and tele-diagnostic, teleconsultation and tele-treatment and tele-education and teleconsultation [30].

Teledentistry has yet to be employed as a routine delivery system. Wider implementation would also require appropriate health policies and strategies, as well as political support for these initiatives. In many countries, teledentistry initiatives are behind e-health progress. Also, there is a need to expand the evidence on which decisions to implement teledentistry programmes are based. For example, in Australia, there are Medicare benefits available for teleconsultation between medical specialists and patients who are located in telehealth eligible areas. They are also available in eligible aged care facilities and Aboriginal medical services throughout Australia [41]. Medicare benefits are also available for clinical support provided by a health professional who is with the patient during the video consultation [41]. However, so far, dentistry is not included in this scheme.

1.4 Towards e-Oral Health as a Scientific Field of Inquiry

However, while Mariño and Ghanim concluded that teledentistry is a mature field, more information about the implementation of clinical uses is still needed [30]. Teledentistry solutions require rigorous evaluation to inform policies and strategies on ICT and telehealth applications in oral health. This will create new opportunities to support, promote and facilitate research and projects that use ICT tools and technologies for the improvement of oral health. There is also a need for more studies and information on the economic benefits of telemedicine, in particular, teledentistry solutions. Legal and ethical considerations also need to be addressed, as well as policies on data transferring and confidentiality.

Furthermore, a report from Ernst and Young identified six megatrends, each of them standing on its own but with a clear interactivity. These include a digital future, rising entrepreneurship, a global market place, an increasingly urbanised world, a resourceful planet and reimagined health [8]. These trends are driving a fundamentally different approach to the delivery of health care. These developments will lead to a chain of interconnected pieces of information from a "single molecule to the entire human population" [42]. For this to happen, a new generation of oral health scientists who can combine knowledge and skills from clinical and public health research and informatics is required [43].

Kuhn and his collaborators [42] group this research challenges into four areas: bioinformatics and systems biology, biomedical engineering and informatics, health informatics and individual health care and public health informatics. A recently created network within the International Association for Dental Research in e-oral health creates a forum and opportunities to support, promote and facilitate research, best clinical and public health practices and educational and learning programmes that use ICT tools and technologies for the improvement of oral health. The network, through its various activities and members, will assist in the promotion and dissemination of e-health research and evidence of teledentistry and telehealth outcomes, as well as generate cooperation and research between experts in the areas of informatics, engineering, economics, statistics and social sciences.

While the field of teledentistry is growing and developing in a consistent fashion, teledentistry cannot provide the complete answer to everything; however, it will never realise its full potential if it does not receive the attention it deserves. Given current technological trends, and the number and magnitude of changes brought by ICT, its potential applications will only increase in the future and will be implemented in an increasing number of countries around the world. Thus, it can be expected that teledentistry will follow the patterns in research output that characterise the trends in the field of telemedicine. Future cooperation with the public sector and research will make available the benefits of new technologies in ICT. This will drive a reduction in health inequalities and improve access to health as a human right, improving quality of life and social participation. Nonetheless, while the use of ICT by the public is wide, its access is still not universal. Access to telemedicine is so far unequal within and between countries [44].

On the other hand, it is essential that practitioners and the public grasp these technologies to reach their full potential. Oral health professionals must be trained in the use of teledentistry. It is assumed that today's oral health professionals and students are computer literate. However, this needs to be further explored, as it may still be the case that a digital divide exists among the future oral health workforce [45]. Thus, more needs to be done at dental schools or in continued professional development courses to prepare oral health professional for the use of this technology.

Conclusions

In many countries considerable inequalities exist in access to health-care services; income level, geographical location and cultural distance are among these barriers. Teledentistry seeks to provide and/or support oral health care in areas underserved by dental practitioners, transcending these barriers. Teledentistry has the potential to reduce costs, improve patient outcomes and deliver greater access to quality dental care. Teledentistry can benefit oral health care by enhancing early diagnosis, facilitating timely treatment of oral diseases, reducing isolation of practitioners through communication with peers and consultation with specialists and improving access to care.

Information and communications technology (ICT) has been used in medicine for over 40 years for diagnosis, consultation and treatment. Telemedicine already has considerable impact on the health-care industry to deliver health records, graphics, audio and digital imaging between participants who are physically at a distance from one another for the purpose of communication enhancement and oral health-care improvement and education. Teledentistry, when compared to medicine, is a relatively new area of health using ICT. Nonetheless, if dentistry parallels medicines, the implementation of teledentistry will occur in various institutions and organisations around the world, including low- and middle-income countries. People living in rural or underserved areas are among those that will most benefit from ICT uses in dentistry.

However, for teledentistry to be an effective oral health-care model which incorporates evidence-based approaches, it needs to expand beyond pilot and field tests. It is also important that all sites involved are adequately resourced in terms of staff, equipment, telecommunications, technical support and training. In particular, training for teledentistry operators is essential. Users should be trained in the use of the equipment and have access to technical support to troubleshoot any difficulties. Furthermore, training and research are important factors in the successful implementation of teledentistry solutions. More research is needed to establish the evidence base to support teledentistry practice. Thus, this chapter's aim is to provide the foundation for teledentistry and underline its merits for the delivery of oral health care. The chapter also discusses the opportunities and benefits associated with the adoption of teledentistry solutions as well as its utilisation and impact on the oral health system and the population.

References

1. Lahanas M. Ancient Greek communication methods. Available at http://www.mlahanas.de/Greeks/Communication.htm. Accessed 27 June 2016.
2. Bashshur R, Shannon GW. History of telemedicine: evolution, context, and transformation. New Rochelle: Mary Ann Liebert; 2009.
3. Zundel KM. Telemedicine: history, applications, and impact on librarianship. Bull Med Libr Assoc. 1996;84:71–9.
4. Vladzymyrskyy A, Jordanova M, Lievens F. A century of telemedicine: Curatio Sine Distantia et Tempora. Sofia: Malina Jordanova; 2016.
5. Eikelboom RH. The telegraph and the beginnings of telemedicine in Australia. Stud Health Technol Inform. 2012;182:67–72.
6. Acierno L. The history of cardiology. N Engl J Med. 1995;332:129–30.
7. Iafolla T. History of telemedicine infographic. 2016. Available at https://evisit.com/history-telemedicine-infographic/. Accessed 24 June 2016.
8. Ernst and Young. Megatrends 2015: making sense of a world in motion. 2015. Available at http://www.ey.com/GL/en/Issues/Business-environment/ey-megatrends-that-will-shape-our-future-4-global-marketplace. Accessed 24 June 2016.
9. Standards Australia. What is health informatics? 2016. Available at http://www.e-health.standards.org.au/ABOUTIT014/WhatisHealthInformatics.aspx. Accessed 23 June 2016.
10. Pan American Health Organization (PAHO). Strategy and plan of action on eHealth. CD51/13 (Eng.). 2011. Available at http://iris.paho.org/xmlui/handle/123456789/1721/. Accessed 29 June 2016.
11. World Health Organization. WHO library cataloguing-in-publication data telemedicine: opportunities and developments in member states: report on the second global survey on eHealth 2009. Global observatory for eHealth series, vol. 2. 2010. Available at http://www.who.int/goe/publications/ehealth_series_vol2/en/. Accessed 30 June 2016.

12. European Commission. E-health - making healthcare better for European citizens: an action plan for a European eHealth area. 2004. Available at http://eur-ex.europa.eu/LexUriServ/LexUriServ.do?uri=COM:2004:0356:FIN:EN:PDF. Accessed 26 June 2016.
13. Cook J, Austen G, Stephens C. Videoconferencing: what are the benefits for dental practice? Br Dent J. 2000;188:67–70.
14. Chen JW, Hobdell MH, Dunn K, Johnson KA, Zhang J. Teledentistry and its use in dental education. J Am Dent Assoc. 2003;134:342–6.
15. Brüllmann D, Schmidtmann I, Warzecha K, d'Hoedt B. Recognition of root canal orifices at a distance—a preliminary study of teledentistry. J Telemed Telecare. 2011;17:154–7.
16. Birnbach JM. The future of teledentistry. J Calif Dent Assoc. 2000;28:141–3.
17. Mea VD. Prerecorded telemedicine. J Telemed Telecare. 2005;11:276–84.
18. Sanchez Dils E, Lefebvre C, Abeyta K. Teledentistry in the United States: a new horizon of dental care. Int J Dent Hyg. 2004;2:161–4.
19. Mariño R, Tonmukayakul U, Marwaha P, Collmann R, Hopcraft M, Manton D, Stranieri A, Clarke K. Teleconsultation/telediagnosis using teledentistry technology: a pilot feasibility study. Int J Adv Life Sci. 2014;6:291–9.
20. Cook J. ISDN video conferencing in postgraduate dental education and orthodontic diagnosis. In: learning technology in medical education conference 1997 (CTI Medicine). 1997. p. 111–116.
21. Curtis EK. Exploring teledentistry. AGD Impact. 2009;37:34.
22. Joshi V. Teledentistry: e-consultations. Dentistry Magazine. 9 February 2002. 2000. Available at http://www.dental-consults.com/dentistry.html. Accessed 24 June 2016.
23. Berndt J, Leone P, King G. Using teledentistry to provide interceptive orthodontic services to disadvantaged children. Am J Orthod Dentofac Orthop. 2008;134:700–6.
24. Chang SW, Plotkin DR, Mulligan R, Polido JC, Mah JK, Meara JG. Teledentistry in rural California: a USC initiative. J Calif Dent Assoc. 2003;31:601–8.
25. Manning D. Florida state oral health improvement plan (SOHIP) teledentistry workgroup chair, in the 2006 Florida Department of Health White Paper Teledentistry as a method to improve oral health access in Florida. 2006.
26. Daniel SJ, Kumar S. Teledentistry: a key component in access to care. J Evid Based Dent Pract. 2014;14:S201–8.
27. Clark GT. Teledentistry: what is it now, and what will it be tomorrow? J Calif Dent Assoc. 2000;28:121–7.
28. Bauer JC, Brown WT. The digital transformation of oral health care: teledentistry and electronic commerce. J Am Dent Assoc. 2001;132:204–9.
29. American Dental Association. ADA center for informatics and standards. What is dental informatics?. 2016. Available at http://www.ada.org/en/member-center/member-benefits/practice-resources/dental-informatics. Accessed 24 June 2016.
30. Mariño R, Ghanim A. Teledentistry: a systematic review of the literature. J Telemed Telecare. 2013;19:179–83.
31. Salley JJ, Zimmerman JL, Ball MJ. Dental informatics: what, why, who, where, and when. In: Dental informatics: strategic issues for the dental profession, Lecture notes in medical informatics, vol. 39. Berlin: Springer-Verlag; 1990. p. 1–6.
32. Rocca MA, Kudryk VL, Pajak JC, Morris T. The evolution of a teledentistry system within the Department of Defense. Proc AMIA Symp. 1999:921–4.
33. Allukian M Jr. The neglected epidemic and the surgeon general's report: a call to action for better oral health. Am J Public Health. 2008;98:S82–5.
34. Beetstra S, Derksen D, Ro M, Powell W, Fry DE, Kaufman A. A "health commons" approach to oral health for low-income populations in a rural state. Am J Public Health. 2008;98:S89–90.
35. Armer JM. A case study of the use of telemedicine by advanced practice nurses in rural Missouri. J Contin Educ Nurs. 2003;34:226–33.
36. Fricton J, Chen H. Using teledentistry to improve access to dental care for the underserved. Dent Clin N Am. 2009;53:537–48.

37. Mariño R, Manton D, Marwaha P, Hallett K, Clarke K, Hopcraft M, McCullough M, Borda A. The implementation of paediatric teledentistry. Global Health 2014. 2014. Available at http://www.thinkmind.org/index.php?view=article&articleid=global_health_2014_1_40_70098. Accessed 28 June 2016.
38. Mariño R, Hopcraft M, Collmann R, Manton D, McCullough M, Clarke K, Ozanne E, Blackberry I. A teledentistry approach for oral health screening in nursing homes. International Federation on Ageing 11th Global Conference. Prague, 2012. 2012. Available at http://www.ifa-fiv.org/wp-content/uploads/2013/12/Marino-Rodrigo-A-Teledentistry-Approach-for-Oral-Health-Screening-in-Nursing-Home.pdf. Accessed 24 June 2016.
39. Torres-Pereira C, Possebon RS, Simões A, Bortoluzzi MC, Leão JC, Giovanini AF, Piazetta CM. Email for distance diagnosis of oral diseases: a preliminary study of teledentistry. J Telemed Telecare. 2008;14:435–8.
40. Younai FS, Messadi DV. E-mail-based oral medicine consultation. J Calif Dent Assoc. 2000;28:144–51.
41. Australian Department of Human Services. Telehealth and medicare benefits schedule. 2016. Available at https://www.humanservices.gov.au/health-professionals/services/medicare/mbs-and-telehealth. Accessed 27 June 2016.
42. Kuhn KA, Knoll A, Mewes HW, Schwaiger M, Bode A, Broy M, Daniel H, Feussner H, Gradinger R, Hauner H, Höfler H, Holzmann B, Horsch A, Kemper A, Krcmar H, Kochs EF, Lange R, Leidl R, Mansmann U, Mayr EW, Meitinger T, Molls M, Navab N, Nüsslin F, Peschel C, Reiser M, Ring J, Rummeny EJ, Schlichter J, Schmid R, Wichmann HE, Ziegler S. Informatics and medicine: from molecules to populations. Methods Inf Med. 2008;47:283–95.
43. Altman RB, Balling R, Brinkley JF, Coiera E, Consorti F, Dhansay MA, Geissbuhler A, Hersh W, Kwankam SY, Lorenzi NM, Martin-Sanchez F, Mihalas GI, Shahar Y, Takabayashi K, Wiederhold G. Commentaries on "Informatics and medicine: from molecules to populations". Methods Inf Med. 2008;47:296–317.
44. Research 2 Guidance. European countries are behind the USA in regards to telemedicine maturity, but they're beginning to catch up - research2guidance. 2015. Available at http://research2guidance.com/2015/11/10/european-countries-are-behind-the-usa-in-regards-to-telemedicine-maturity-but-theyre-beginning-to-catch-up/. Accessed 30 June 2016.
45. Mariño R, Habibi E, Au-Yeung W, Morgan M. Use of communication and information technology among Victorian and South Australian oral health profession students. J Dent Educ. 2012;76:1667–74.

e-Oral Health Tools

2

Rodrigo Mariño and Alagesan Chinnasamy

Abstract

Telemedicine has been in use for over 30 years for consultation, diagnosis and treatment, in a broad range of medical fields; despite this, there has been little use of similar ICT-focused practices within oral health. Notwithstanding the relatively slow adoption of teledentistry, the application of ICT in dentistry is increasing. The application of teledentistry suggests a range of possible beneficial applications, such as the efficient delivery of health records, improved communication between providers and patients and enhanced education opportunities. This chapter describes the main e-oral health tools already available for practitioners. It presents the limitations and advantages which need to be taken into consideration. The chapter also notes the non-ICT tools necessary for wider implementation, including legal, ethical and regulation challenges. For teledentistry to be effective, it is also important that all sites involved are adequately resourced in terms of staff, equipment, telecommunications, technical support and training. Enabling tools covered in this chapter also include organisational change and the development of user friendly e-oral health systems, as well as new skills among oral health practitioners.

Keywords

e-oral health • Teledentistry • e-tools

R. Mariño (✉) • A. Chinnasamy
Melbourne Dental School, The University of Melbourne, Melbourne, 3010 Victoria, Australia
e-mail: r.marino@unimelb.edu.au

N. Giraudeau (ed.), *e-Health Care in Dentistry and Oral Medicine*,
https://doi.org/10.1007/978-3-319-69450-4_2

2.1 Introduction

Despite the rapid advancement of science and technology in the last century, it was not until its last decades that those advancements took over, fundamentally modifying how dentistry is practised and regulated [1]. As described in the previous chapter, technological advancements in the last few years have driven the massive adoption and use of information and communications technology (ICT) by the general population, as well as the development of e-health tools, creating new solutions including products, systems and services that go beyond simple Internet-based applications.

There is widespread use of applications (Apps) with the ubiquitous presence of Internet and mobile technology. e-Tools can be defined as a computer- or web-based application intended to make a task easier. Examples of e-tools include health information networks, electronic health records, telemedicine services, personal wearable, portable communicable systems, health portals and many other applications used in health care for monitoring, prevention, early detection, diagnosis and management of diseases or conditions. In some respects, telehealth devices are not different to old equipment but smaller with greater scope of features. Having said that, they are not just a mere replacement of existing tools to deliver the same outcome. These advancements represent a new paradigm, allowing for opportunities for features that were not available before. They transform equipment and models at a deeper level, creating networks, sending information, tracking performance and remote monitoring of participants. This would mean reduced costs, improved patient outcomes and greater access to quality oral health care. The whole community will ultimately benefit from this transformation.

These days, e-health tools include tools for health authorities, for health professionals, as well as personalised health systems for patients and the general public [2]. For patients, the use of ICT in oral health seeks to provide and/or support dental care in areas underserved by dental practitioners, transcending social, geographic and cultural barriers. e-Health tools also empowered health consumers. From the providers' side, e-health tools can make fast and easy access to e-records and to images anywhere, and a telehealth solution would also take less time as it avoids time spent commuting. e-Referrals and e-prescriptions increase the speed of access and decrease mistakes [3]. For health authorities, advances in technology for new diagnostic tools and therapeutic procedures, together with demographic changes in the population, are escalating the cost of health care, including oral health care [4]. Within this context, biomedical informatics and teledentistry have the potential to reduce costs, improve patient outcomes and offer greater access to quality oral health care, even in real time [4].

Furthermore, tools also include the development of new skills; organisational changes; regulation frameworks; measures to ensure safety; finances; and technical issues (e.g. interconnectivity), as e-health solutions cannot be an independent piece. Apart from regulation, there are also ethical issues to consider. Thus, when all combined, e-health tools can help respond to the major challenges of the health sector, by facilitating the delivery of better health care, with reduced cost and improved patient-centred health delivery systems.

This chapter presents an overview of the many ICT and e-tools available for oral health, their limitations and advantages. The chapter is organised into two main

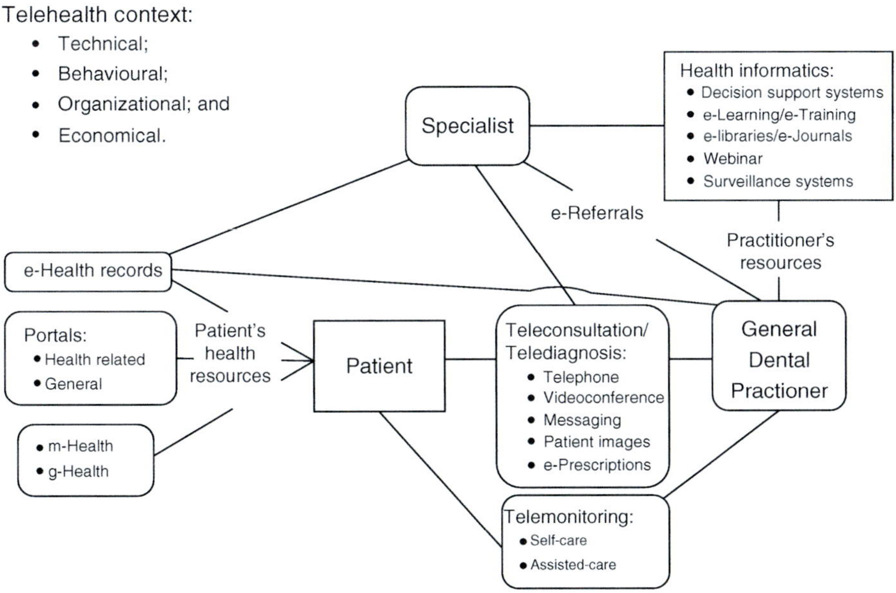

Fig. 2.1 e-Oral health tools framework

sections; the first section will look at e-oral health tools for patients, oral health professionals and health managers. As teledentistry services would involve multiple roles and players, the second section will address additional arrangement including challenges for implementation of those e-tools for oral health. This includes technical, behavioural, organisational and economic and finances tools. The framework used in this chapter is presented in Fig. 2.1.

2.2 Tools for e-Oral Health and Teledentistry

Some of the uses of e-health include the delivery of health services using ICT, comprising mobile health (mHealth), electronic records, tele-education, tele-training, eLearning for distance learning, tele-monitoring, telediagnosis, teleconsultation and e-distribution of oral health promotion and health education. e-Health also includes tele-support to remote health facilities located in isolated areas, remote places or in areas affected by natural disasters or armed conflict. More recently, gamification, or gHealth, is also becoming a powerful tool in health care. gHealth allows rewards for individuals that follow the regime, as an engagement mechanism.

2.2.1 Teleconsultation and Telediagnosis

An oral health screening can be performed by a telehealth assistant to an oral health professional at a distant site, thus reducing the need for an oral health professional (or the patient) to travel to health-care facilities, particularly those located in rural areas. A teledentistry consultation begins much like a conventional face-to-face oral health consultation. The local general dental practitioner (GDP) or oral health professional or other trained personnel collect information about patient's medical and oral health histories. Then a live consultation may be conducted with the clinician at the remote expert site or the collected information along with videos and photographs captured using the intraoral camera forwarded electronically to the oral health professional for review of the received materials, leading to referral and treatment recommendations.

With the exception of the intraoral camera, much of the equipment required for teledentistry may already be available as they are used for other functions and can be shared if planned appropriately. The technology required for teledentistry is not complex, comprising hardware, software and Internet connectivity. The hardware comprises a computer, or tablet, that has reasonable hard drive storage (greater than 250 GB) and a substantial amount of random access memory (RAM) coupled with a processer able to handle real-time video processing along with a web camera for videoconferencing and an intraoral dental camera to capture images. Finally, sufficient bandwidth is required to support the desired consultation model: real time or store and forward [5].

When looking at technical advantages, the intraoral camera produces images that are as good as or superior to visual examination. Thus, there is potential to improve the diagnosis of oral diseases, in particular, dental caries, as it has been reported that teledentistry enhances the detection of active dental caries [6]. However, because a hands-on examination cannot be performed, the specialist must depend on the information from the examination carried out at the remote site. Confidence and good cooperative relationships between team members at both sites must be established [7].

2.2.2 Monitoring Applications

Of all the e-health tools, mHealth, with the use of applications (Apps) and gHealth, seems to be progressing at the fastest pace. In fact, today, more people have access to a mobile phone than to clean drinking water, toilet or electricity [8]. mHealth is regarded as a subset of e-health, and its domain is the medical or public health practice supported by mobile devices. Health-related Apps are increasing at a high speed. Most are designed to monitor aspect of an individual's health profile and status. Mobile Apps are software written to run on smartphones, tablets and other mobile devices.

Biometric measuring devices, such as heart rate, blood pressure, glucose level, etc., come under the health monitoring systems (HMS) and use a range of technological devices to remotely monitor the health and clinical signs of a patient. Because HMS mostly use store and forward, they are able to overcome the limitations of face-to-face delivery, such as time constraints, access issues, availability and cost. As with all types of monitoring systems, the aims of HMS are to detect activities of daily living, occurrence of significant events (i.e. falls), changes in health status or a combination of these [9]. Monitoring is an example of secondary prevention applications. HMS can be further broken down to:

- Wearable health monitoring systems (WHMS): wearable devices or biosensors that can be worn by patients. Examples of these are smart vests where a variety of sensors are integrated into the garment's fabric [10]. These sensors can simultaneously collect bio-signals in a non-invasive and unobtrusive way to measure cardiac parameters [9]. Wearable salivary uric acid mouth-guard biosensors are used to measure uric acid levels in saliva for kidney disease and diabetes [11]. WHMS are used to detect falls in elderly [8], and they can also be used to help monitor and prevent severe adverse effects of orofacial trauma in older adults and children with special needs.
- Mobile health monitoring systems. Mobile technology, such as smartphone applications, can be used to manage and track health conditions or promote healthy behaviours. For example, they are used in health-care services to send automatic reminders to patients such as e-mails, SMS, etc. to confirm appointments [12]. They are found to be more convenient and cost-effective than traditional, institutional care, since they enable patients to remain in their usual environment while receiving professional health care [13]. This could include Apps that monitor patient toothbrushing or other home care and smart toothbrushes.
- Remote health monitoring systems can benefit people living in underserved areas (i.e. residential aged care faculties) and those living in rural and remote areas with limited access to health care in the management of chronic diseases, such as cardiovascular disease, diabetes mellitus and asthma. The patient's health information is gathered through technological devices and sent for evaluation and stored in the patient's medical records for future use.

There are many outstanding Apps to help people improve their health. However, there are also some warnings about them. For example, while many Apps contain sound medical information, medical diagnostic equipment is highly specialised and specific. An App does not put a general medical practitioner or a specialist medical lab in your pocket. They are no substitute for a consultation with a general medical practitioner or specialist. Human involvement has to be kept in the loop. Thus, App development needs to involve both public health and clinical professionals who are able to address the health problem of the patient. This will lead to better results and much higher acceptance, for both the patient and the professional.

2.2.3 Smart Glass as an Oral Health Clinical Tool

Smart glasses are becoming popular among GDPs [14]. The technology incorporates a head-mounted display and computer that is designed to allow the wearer real-time Internet access, communications, audio/video/photo and research capabilities. In addition, a live feed to smart glass would provide an excellent solution to displaying remote clinical and patient information, which also makes smart glasses an important tool for local dentists seeking support from metro-based specialists.

For example, the clinician could view X-rays and 3-D scans via smart glass while performing procedures and/or be guided by a remote expert to improve outcomes.

2.2.4 Personally Controlled e-Records

The progression of e-health and the personally controlled electronic health record (PCEHR) offers great opportunities for sharing critical health information between health professionals and the patient [2]. Furthermore, the use of e-record would also allow for research, public health information and health data to be easily available. They are also important as they increase the speed of access and minimising error [3].

2.2.5 e-Tools for Primary Prevention

Teledentistry and e-health solutions have the potential to be highly effective mechanisms for enhancing early diagnosis and referral for patients who otherwise might not receive care. Monitoring and screening are frequently used for secondary prevention through store and forward. e-Health solutions in preventive health are less developed than curative health. Nonetheless, there is an enormous potential for e-tool solutions to provide more accessible and effective e-heath solutions, particularly in primary prevention. Primary prevention solutions will help individuals stay healthy, or how to monitor risk factors for disease in the community. This takes us to an emerging phenomenon: the empowered, independent and networked consumer.

2.2.5.1 Gamification (gHealth)

Gamification is the application of game elements and digital game design techniques to everyday problems such as business dilemmas and social challenges [15]. gHealth includes novel ways to promote healthy behaviours and behavioural change using social media, gaming and multimedia and several game designs to affect behaviour change in at-risk groups, for training and education, getting people involved in new ideas and gaining feedback for the community. Games can be used to transmit adherence data, which would allow for resources to be targeted, for example, to those who are non-compliant. It allows for rewards to individuals that follow the regime, as an engagement mechanism.

The result is the development of game concepts that are engaging, instructionally relevant and accessible across a wide variety of delivery platforms, including Facebook, web sites, mobile gaming, CD-ROM and gaming consoles [15].

2.2.5.2 Web Portals

A web portal is a site in the WWW that functions as a point of access to information, resources and databases. A portal presents information from several sources. Portals hosted by government or responsible institutions are sources. Table 2.1 shows some selected general health and oral health portals prompting healthy behaviours.

Table 2.1 General and oral health portals

General health portal
• Centers for Disease Control and Prevention: http://www.cdc.gov/
• World Health Organization: http://www.who.int/en/
• Health-EU portal: http://ec.europa.eu/health/index_en.htm
• WebMD: http://www.webmd.com/
• National Institutes of Health: https://www.nih.gov/
• Medscape: http://www.medscape.com/
• Health Info: http://www.healthinfonet.ecu.edu.au/
• National Health Service: http://www.nhs.uk
• Patient Info: www.patient.co.uk
• Canada Health: http://www.hc-sc.gc.ca/index-eng.php
• Surgeon General: http://www.surgeongeneral.gov/
• Healthdirect: http://www.healthinsite.gov.au
Oral health portal
• Oral Health CRC http://www.oralhealthcrc.org.au/
• British Dental Health Foundation: https://www.dentalhealth.org/
• World Health Organization Oral Health: http://www.who.int/oral_health/en/
• Centers for Disease Control and Prevention Oral health: http://www.cdc.gov/oralhealth/

2.3 Arrangement for Wider Implementation of e-Oral Health and Teledentistry

e-Health has become common place for health professionals, patients and the community. Nonetheless, teledentistry solutions need to incorporate service delivery systems to address the identified demand for oral health care for underserved populations in nontraditional settings. There is a need for new tools, definitions and standards, as well as ensuring that the organisation fits the new service rather than making the technology fit the old organisation [16]. Barriers for the diffusion of telehealth can be grouped within four categories, as delineated by Tanriverdi and Iacono [17]: technical, behavioural, organisational and economical.

2.3.1 Technical

The development of fast, cheap and reliable Internet connections will allow for good two-way interactive communication and will open a broad range of opportunities. Broadband networks, such as the National Broadband Network in Australia, enable access to technology and information and provide enormous potential to offer more accessible and effective e-health solutions. Still, even when there are areas with low speed connectivity, some e-health solutions can work reasonably well using store and forward [3], particularly when good-quality two-way interaction between a service provider and a patient is not required. Remote and isolated areas of a country are the most likely to benefit from enhancements in connectivity.

Interoperability issues with telemedicine and teledentistry.

It is not uncommon to see health information being recorded electronically, or on paper and sometimes a combination of both, but held in different locations. This can pose a problem as it becomes difficult to gain a complete understanding of the patient health-care journey. Different health-care professionals have their own procedures and health information systems (HIS). The general practitioner (GP) has the GP-HIS, the community nurse has community HIS, and health-care workers in hospitals use hospital HIS [18]. Further complicating the issues, there is sometimes disintegration or fragmentation of services within the public health-care system [19]. These issues can lead to miscommunication or missing patient information, ultimately compromising patient safety.

Interoperability enables seamless integration of systems and software applications to communicate, exchange data and work together within and across organisational boundaries, using the information to advance health status and the effective delivery of health care for individuals and communities [20]. This depends on standardisation of components and services. Thus, a consideration for developers is the construct of a solution with interoperability standards. For example, standards such as HL7 and CEN/ISO 1360 would help overcome many of these challenges by making data sharing across clinicians, lab, hospital, pharmacy and patients easier [21].

2.3.2 Behavioural

When planning the range of skills necessary in the future health workforce, in addition to clinical skills, the workforce will need to develop skills in information technology, health education and communication [22]. Training is a very important factor for success [23]. A teledentistry system will be underused if the patient information exists but the connection is ineffectual, either for technical reasons or because the suitable staff are not available at the diagnostic end. For teledentistry to be effective, it is also important that all sites involved are adequately resourced in terms of staff, equipment, telecommunications, technical support and training. In particular, training for teledentistry operators is essential, as other nonclinicians are also part of the successful implementation. The operator should be familiar with the use of computer technology in order to be efficient enough to absorb instructions easily and thus overcome the time factor [24]. The operator also needs confidence around basic concepts and tools required for teledentistry consultations and to allow practitioners with little or no formal training or experience in oral health to enter into this process. Therefore, it is important to ensure that there is an adequately trained team to enable links to be used with minimum delays, even in emergencies [25].

To practise dentistry, regardless of your professional background or specialty, oral health professionals rely on continuous update of the body of information that is developed in laboratories, clinical and community trials, etc. In fact, oral health professionals are taught that a substantial proportion of the material covered in dental schools will become obsolete within a few years. Keeping abreast with technical and literature is an obligation expected from an oral health professional. Evidence-based practice (EBP) and critical thinking are essential skills for the oral health professionals. There is an urgent need for oral health professionals to use research to inform their practice. No practitioner can be a competent and effective health provider without knowing how to read and critically evaluate the ever-changing and rapidly evolving research knowledge that is being generated and presented in the modern online space. These days, sharing of research and information has become easier. Methods of sharing information are increasing with open access journals, digital libraries and social networks.

Academic institutions have a role in training oral health professionals to develop an educational strategy on telehealth training and education. One approach to these challenges is to change the structure of how we train oral health students, how we model the interaction GDP/patient and management of health [26], and also how students and oral health professionals gather, organise and use information in their professional life.

2.3.3 Organisational

2.3.3.1 Sustainability and Institutionalisation

Teledentistry schemes, so far, have generally made only the initial steps towards institutionalisation and are seen by health authorities and the dental profession in general as pilot research projects, funded by research grants [27]. Thus, full implementation and institutionalisation may take longer and require additional tools.

For true self-sustainability and institutionalisation, a telehealth programme cannot depend on altruistic tendencies of practitioners/people. By institutionalisation, we refer to the stage when a programme 'settles' into an organisation and becomes 'embedded' into its normal activities. It becomes part of the organisation hierarchy and standard operations and procedures, with a dedicated annual budget, etc. [28]. The process leading to institutionalisation involves several stages. Nonetheless, every telehealth solution must find an adequate revenue model for the practitioner [29].

2.3.3.2 Confidentially, Security and Liability Issues

Regulation Framework

As with any technological advancement in health, new solutions require regulations to ensure privacy, safety and confidentiality. Telehealth has the potential to breach these privileges. The landscape of telehealth and teledentistry is quickly evolving, and regulators need to keep pace with these changes.

The National Committee for Vital and Health Statistics describes privacy as the individual's right to control the acquisition, uses or disclosures of his or her identifiable health data [30]. Confidentiality, which is closely related to privacy, refers to the obligations of those who receive information to respect the privacy interests of those to whom the data relate. On the other hand, security is altogether different; it refers to physical, technological or administrative safeguards or tools used to protect identifiable health data from unwarranted access or disclosure [30]. These concerns arise from the transfer of medical histories and records as well as from general security issues of electronic information stored in computers. Concerns may also arise about the proper method of informing patients of the potential risk in the transmission of their data [31]. There is a lack of control or limits on the data collection of personal information. For instance, home sensors intended to detect falls, that may very well include some dental trauma, may also transmit information such as when no one is home [32].

To help overcome some of these issues, technical controls have been developed which can protect against potential security risks [33]. Data encryption is one way of protecting data from being lost to online attackers. This is done using complex mathematical keys, and when attackers gain access, the data becomes meaningless to read. Additional measures to control access to information include authentication of the person's identity [34]. Furthermore, telehealth applications are vulnerable to attacks through malware. Mobile platforms can prevent such malware from being installed on the device [35].

There are also issues around licensure and regulations of oral health professionals who practise teledentistry. A teleconsultation can cross state and even international borders. In this way, an oral health professional can provide advice to a patient or another oral health provider, or even non-health-care providers (e.g. nurse), who would act under this advice. In the USA, an important barrier to a nationwide teledentistry or telemedicine practice is the traditional system of state-by-state licensing, meaning that an oral health professional from one state may not be able to legally provide his or her services via telecommunications to a patient in another state, unless that person is licensed in both states [31]. These state-by-state approaches prevent people from receiving critical, often life-saving medical services that may be available to their neighbours living just across the state line, regardless of whether or not telemedicine is used [36].

As well as legal regulation tasks, there are also ethical issues to solve. These include the three principles or ethical standards to be observed: respect for persons, protecting the autonomy of all people; beneficence, maximising benefits while minimising risks to people; and justice, ensuring reasonable, nonexploitative and well-considered procedures are administered with fair distribution of costs and benefits to potential participants.

2.3.4 Economical

Related to the ethical principle of justice is the demand for resources to be equitably distributed [36]. Reimbursement mechanisms have to be revised with telehealth in mind [37]. For example, in Australia, there are Medicare benefits available for teleconsultation between medical specialists and patients who are located in telehealth eligible areas. They are also available in eligible aged care facilities and Aboriginal medical services throughout Australia. Medicare benefits are also available for clinical support provided by a health professional who is with the patient during the video consultation. However, so far, dentistry is not included in this scheme. On the other hand, in November 2015, The American Dental Association House of

Delegates passed a resolution which states that dental benefit plans and other third-party payers, public and private programmes, should cover services provided through teledentistry at the same level as if the services were delivered in a traditional in-person encounter [38]. Within Europe, Norway became an ideal setting for telemedicine including teledentistry because of the scattered population and scarcity of health services in the northern region. In 1996, Norway also became the first country to implement an official telemedicine fee schedule making telemedicine services reimbursable by the national health insurer [39].

A telehealth solution must ensure confidence, convenience and compensation for its users [29]. It should not create more risk to the patient or increase the practitioner's risk of legal and financial liabilities [28]. Teledentistry and telemedicine both raise concerns about liability, and while there is a lot to consider, such as state laws, payment issues and licensing regulations to practice, liability is often overlooked by health practitioners but may carry the bigger risk [40]. Regarding financial liabilities, the telehealth solution should take less time; if it takes more time, it has to compensate elsewhere, for example, if the practitioner can avoid the time spent going to and from hospitals to see patients [28].

2.4 Final Remarks

Teledentistry will continue to evolve; its advantages may be especially beneficial in remote and rural areas or in underserved populations. Other applications include connecting regions with limited infrastructure with specialists to improve care. Wider implementation would require appropriate health policies and strategies, as well as political support, for these initiatives. Still, many countries are behind in e-health progress. Similarly most countries do not have clear regulations governing telemedicine parity [41].

Oral health programmes are essential for countries' ability to maximise the impact of the health sector in reaching national health objectives and/or priorities and meeting health and social challenges. Teledentistry is about the provision of access to oral heath to populations who otherwise might not receive oral health care. While certain precautions must be made when determining the scope of practice and supervision to nonclinicians and allied health personnel, our ethical obligation is to use tools to reach populations who are unable to receive oral health care. From this perspective, it may be unethical to deprive these populations of oral health care [37]. As individuals and professionals, the challenge is to equip ourselves to be part of the successful resolution of barriers to care, and teledentistry can bring a reduction of oral health inequalities. Access to health is a human right; by facilitating access to technology and information, e-health has proven to be a means for enhancing oral health status, social participation and the quality of life of the population. Consequently, e-oral health is essential for achieving the UN Sustainable Development Goals (SDG) [42] particularly SDG3 ('Ensure healthy lives and promoting well-being for all at all ages'). Additionally, almost all of the other 16 non-health goals are directly related to health or will contribute to health indirectly [43].

Given the current technological trends and the number and magnitude of changes brought by ICT, its potential applications in oral health will only increase. They are already becoming a significant part of oral health care. While oral health professionals cannot treat the majority of dental problems by teleconsultation or telediagnosis, teledentistry nevertheless has the potential to be a highly effective mechanism for enhancing early diagnosis and referral for patients who otherwise might not receive oral health care. This chapter has covered the main e-oral health tools already available for practitioners, that is, advancements that already exist, no new technology is required, and although at present nobody can rely on diagnostic computer programmes, the introduction of new e-health initiatives is making these options even more viable.

Conclusion

In this chapter we present many e-tools of importance, as well as their limitations and advantages which need to be taken into consideration. Telehealth will continue to evolve with advances in ICT. This growth will guide future development of e-tools with new technologies, applications and innovative service delivery methods. For example, telepresence may allow for remote treatment via e-health devices. This might sound like science fiction, but it can be a reality in the future. However, wider implementation also faces legal, ethical and regulatory challenges, which would require appropriate health policies and strategies to address these issues, as well as political support for these initiatives. In many countries, these health policies and strategies are behind e-health progress, including less middle-income countries [44]. It is also necessary to expand the evidence on which we base decisions as well as address the lack of regulation and fragmentation of systems.

References

1. Rocca MA, Kudryk VL, Pajak JC, Morris T. The evolution of a teledentistry system within the Department of Defense. Proc AMIA Symp. 1999:921–4.
2. Ernst and Young. Making sense of a world in motion. 2015. Available from http://www.ey.com/Publication/vwLUAssets/ey-megatrends-report-2015/$FILE/ey-megatrends-report-2015.pdf.
3. Pietrzak E, Pullman S, Cotea C, Nasveld P, Warfe P. How will the introduction of the national broadband network change the face of preventive medicine? e-Health Research Unit. Centre for Military & Veterans' Health. 2011.
4. Kuhn K, Knoll A, Mewes H, Schwaiger M, Bode A, Broy M, et al. From molecules to populations. Methods Inf Med. 2008;47(4):283–95.
5. Mariño R, Manton D, Hopcraft M, McCullough M, Hallett K, Clarke K, et al. Paediatric teledentistry: delivering oral health services to rural and regional children. 2014. Available from: http://networkedsociety.unimelb.edu.au/__data/assets/pdf_file/0019/1661320/Paediatric-Teledentisty.pdf.
6. Kopycka-Kedzierawski DT, Billings RJ, McConnochie KM. Dental screening of preschool children using teledentistry: a feasibility study. Pediatr Dent. 2007;29(3):209–13.
7. Fricton J, Chen H. Using teledentistry to improve access to dental care for the underserved. Dent Clin N Am. 2009;53(3):537–48.
8. United Natiions News Centre. Deputy UN chief calls for urgent action to tackle global

sanitation crisis: United Nations-DPI/NMD - UN News Service Section. 2013. Available from http://www.un.org/apps/news/story.asp?NewsID=44452#.V33FUbh97IX.
9. Peetoom KK, Lexis MA, Joore M, Dirksen CD, De Witte LP. Literature review on monitoring technologies and their outcomes in independently living elderly people. Disabil Rehabil Assist Technol. 2015;10(4):271–94.
10. Pandian P, Mohanavelu K, Safeer K, Kotresh T, Shakunthala D, Gopal P, et al. Smart vest: wearable multi-parameter remote physiological monitoring system. Med Eng Phys. 2008;30(4): 466–77.
11. Kim J, Imani S, de Araujo W, Warchall J, Valdés Ramírez G, Paixão TRLC, et al. Wearable salivary uric acid mouthguard biosensor with integrated wireless electronics. Biosens Bioelectron. 2015;74:1061–8.
12. Daniel H, Sulmasy L. Policy recommendations to guide the use of telemedicine in primary care settings: an American College of Physicians position paper. Ann Intern Med. 2015;163(10):787–9.
13. Tamura T, Togawa T, Ogawa M, Yoda R. Fully automated health monitoring system in the home. Med Eng Phys. 1998;20(8):573–9.
14. Dental Tribune International. Swiss company develops first Google Glass solution for dentists. 2014. Available from http://www.dental-tribune.com/articles/business/europe/20495_swiss_company_develops_first_google_glass_solution_for_dentists.html.
15. Cummings P, Golson M, Goodman D, Nonamaker L. Gaming to engage the healthcare consumer. 2013. Available from http://www.icfi.com/insights/white-papers/2013/gaming-to-engage-healthcare-consumer.
16. van Dyk L. A review of telehealth service implementation frameworks. Int J Environ Res Public Health. 2014;11:1279–98.
17. Tanriverdi H, Iacono CS. Knowledge barriers to diffusion of telemedicine. In: proceedings of the international conference of the association for information systems, Helsinki, Finland. 1998. p. 39–50.
18. van Velsen L, Solana J, Oude-Nijeweme D'Hollosy W, Garate-Barreiro F, Vollenbroek-Hutten M. Advancing telemedicine services for the aging population: the challenge of interoperability. Stud Health Technol Inform. 2015;217:897–900.
19. Health Information and Quality Authority. Overview of healthcare interoperability standards. 2013. Available from https://www.hiqa.ie/publications/overview-healthcare-interoperability-standards.
20. Healthcare Information and Management Systems Society. What is interoperability?: @ HIMSS. 2016. Available from http://www.himss.org/library/interoperability-standards/what-is-interoperability.
21. American Acadamy of Family Physicians. Interoperability: @aafp. 2013. Available from http://www.aafp.org/advocacy/informed/hit/emr/interoperability.html.
22. Day GE. Is our health workforce prepared for future health megatrends? Aust Health Rev. 2015;39(5):487–8.
23. Harnett B. Telemedicine systems and telecommunications. J Telemed Telecare. 2006;12(1): 4–15.
24. Chen JW, Hobdell MH, Dunn K, Johnson KA, Zhang JJ. Teledentistry and its use in dental education. J Am Dent Assoc. 2003;134(3):342–6.
25. Hoijtink EJ, Rascher I. Telemedicine training & treatment centre "a European rollout of a medical best practice". Stud Health Technol Inform. 2005;114:270.
26. Altman RB, Balling R, Brinkley JF, Coiera E, Consorti F, Dhansay MA, et al. Commentaries on "informatics and medicine: from molecules to populations". Methods Inf Med. 2008;47(4):296–317.
27. Mariño R, Ghanim A. Teledentistry: a systematic review of the literature. J Telemed Telecare. 2013;19(4):179–83.
28. O'Loughlin J, Renaud L, Richard L, Gomez LS, Paradis G. Correlates of the sustainability of community-based heart health promotion interventions. Prev Med. 1998;27(5):702–12.
29. Desai N. Telehealth marketing: the path to patients, profits, and PR. The National Telehealth Webinar Series. The National Network of Telehealth Resource Centers. 2012. Available from

http://www.telehealthresourcecenter.org/sites/main/files/file-attachments/telehealthmarketing_1.pdf.
30. Cohn. The National Committee on Vital and Health Statistics 2006. 2006. Available from http://www.ncvhs.hhs.gov/060622lt.htm.
31. Sfikas PM. Teledentistry: legal and regulatory issues explored. J Am Dent Assoc. 1997;128(12):1716–8.
32. Hall JL, McGraw D. For telehealth to succeed, privacy and security risks must be identified and addressed. Health Aff. 2014;33(2):216–21.
33. Luxton DD, Kayl RA, Mishkind MC. mHealth data security: the need for HIPAA-compliant standardization. Telemed J E Health. 2012;18(4):284–8.
34. Kumar P, Lee S-G, Lee H-J. E-SAP: efficient-strong authentication protocol for healthcare applications using wireless medical sensor networks. Sensors. 2012;12(2):1625–47.
35. National Institute of Standards and Technology. Mobile application vetting services for public safety: National Institute of Standards and Technology. 2016. Available from http://csrc.nist.gov/publications/drafts/nistir-8136/nistir_8136_draft.pdf.
36. Cortez NG, Cohen IG, Kesselheim AS. FDA regulation of mobile health technologies. N Engl J Med. 2014;371(4):372–9.
37. Clark PA, Capuzzi K, Harrison J. Telemedicine: medical, legal and ethical perspectives. Med Sci Monit. 2010;16(12):Ra261–72.
38. American Dental Association. House passes guidelines on teledentistry: American Dental Association. 2015. Available from http://www.ada.org/en/publications/ada-news/2015-archive/december/house-passes-guidelines-on-teledentistry.
39. Hartvigsen G, Johansen MA, Hasvold P, Bellika JG, Arsand E, Arild E, et al. Challenges in telemedicine and eHealth: lessons learned from 20 years with telemedicine in Tromsø. Stud Health Technol Inform. 2007;129(Pt 1):82–6.
40. Gallegos A. Telemedicine poses novel legal risks for doctors: Internal Medicine News. 2015. Available from: http://www.mdedge.com/internalmedicinenews/article/103362/health-policy/telemedicine-poses-novellegal-risks-doctors/page/0/1.
41. Research2guidance. European countries are behind the USA in regards to telemedicine maturity, but they're beginning to catch up - research2guidance: research2guidance. 2015. Updated 10 Nov 2015. Available from http://research2guidance.com/2015/11/10/european-countries-are-behind-the-usa-in-regards-to-telemedicine-maturity-but-theyre-beginning-to-catch-up/.
42. World Health Organization. Health in 2015: from MDGs to SDGs. 2015. Available from http://www.who.int/gho/publications/mdgs-sdgs/en/.
43. Mariño R, Banga RS. UN sustainable development goals (SDGs): a time to act. J Oral Res. 2016;5(1):5–6.
44. Chatzipavlou IA, Christoforidou SA, Vlachopoulou M. A recommended guideline for the development of mHealth apps. mHealth. 2016;2(5):21.

Development of Teledentistry: From Pilot Projects to Successful Implementation

3

Isabelle Bourdon, Roxana Ologeanu-Taddei, and Chris Kimble

Abstract

As of telemedecine initiatives, teledentistry innovations have great potentials to enhance accessibility to dental care, reduce cost of care and enhance quality of dental care. Despite such potentials, many teledentistry innovations remain in the pilot phase or are not successfully implemented. To explain this paradoxe, we discuss the adoption, and the implementation of teledentistry in regular healthcare practices and the evaluation of the success of teledentitry projetc. We propose to identify the main critical factors for teledentistery initiatives.

Keywords

Teledentistry • Healthcare • Innovation

3.1 Introduction

The motivation behind telemedicine initiatives, such as teledentistry, lies in the wish to reduce inequalities in healthcare. Teledentistry, defined as the delivery of dental services through the use of information and communication technologies in a situation where the actors are at different locations, is claimed to improve access to, and the delivery of, oral healthcare while simultaneously decreasing costs [1–4]. Teledentistry is said to be particularly important in rural areas [5] and for those who

I. Bourdon • R. Ologeanu-Taddei (✉)
Montpellier Research Management, Univ. de Montpellier, Montpellier, France
e-mail: isabelle.bourdon@umontpellier.fr; roxana_ologeanu@yahoo.fr

C. Kimble
Montpellier Research Management, Univ. de Montpellier, Montpellier, France
KEDGE Business School, Marseille, France

N. Giraudeau (ed.), *e-Health Care in Dentistry and Oral Medicine*,
https://doi.org/10.1007/978-3-319-69450-4_3

do not have easy access to dental healthcare, such as older people or prisoners [6]. Innovations in teledentistry have the potential to enhance accessibility to dental care, reduce cost of care, and enhance quality of dental care.

These arguments have led healthcare organizations to adopt and implement telemedicine [7] and teledentistry technologies [8] to improve or extend existing patient care and services. Telemedicine and teledentistry represent an important development that has potential for bringing about a paradigmatic shift in healthcare service delivery and collaboration.

Despite such potential, many teledentistry innovations remain in the pilot phase [9] or are not successfully implemented. To explain this fact, we suggest that pilot projects focus on clinical applications and technology development, without taking into account implementation and the critical determinants of a project's success [10]. Pilot projects and clinical experimentation are, in effect, carried out in a controlled environment, while the implementation requires managing the political realities of introducing new technologies into existing organizations, as well as dealing with the financial, organizational, project, and legal implications. For providing support to managers and clinicians aiming to implement large-scale telemedicine projects, we will present in this paper different critical factors for telemedicine projects highlighted by the literature. This paper is structured as follows. Section 3.2 highlights the importance of assessment of pilot projects taking into account different aspects beyond the clinical assessment generally related to a telemedicine project. Section 3.3 briefly presents the importance of the decision to adopt a technology based on pragmatic objectives. Section 3.4 will describe critical factors related to the implementation of the technology as the next step after the adoption decision.

3.2 Assessment of Pilot Projects

The evaluation of the outcomes of pilot projects is generally based on two major frameworks: the framework for the economic evaluation of telemedicine [11] and the model for the assessment of telemedicine (MAST) [12, 13].

Clinical outcomes, either diagnostic accuracy or clinical effectiveness, cost measures, and patient satisfaction were reported frequently in telemedicine studies, but reporting of other performance metrics was rare [9].

Approaches in telemedicine projects' assessment have considered a single evaluation perspective [14]. Multiple assessment dimensions would imply the use of multiple collection and analysis methodologies which will identify the most useful and cost-effective criteria to design and assess a telemedicine application [15]. A three-step model, MAST [13], has been developed for helping organizations to decide whether to implement telemedicine services in healthcare systems and help decision-makers in choosing the most efficient technologies to be used in the most cost-effective way. The focus of the evaluation is the effectiveness of the telemedicine application and was tested by Ekeland and Grøttland [12] in 21 European pilot projects. The MAST model's application in the pilot projects' evaluation revealed some areas that are not covered such as process studies, technological usability, responsible innovation, health literacy, behavior change, caregiver perspectives, and motivational issues of professionals [12]. Moreover, scientific standards and guidelines as bases of assessment seem to be rather difficult to put into practice in some specific areas because such knowledge is not available.

3.3 Decision to Adopt Telemedicine Technology

The adoption of a technology is clearly critical for its utilization and the resultant changes to the level of healthcare provision [7]. The OECD (Value for Money in Health Spending, OECD 2010) considers that the Information Communication Technology can improve patients' safety and efficiency gains, increase compliance with evidence-based guidelines through developing clinical decision systems, and develop telemedicine for rural populations.

Generally, top management of healthcare organizations decide to adopt a telemedicine technology, such as teledentistry, because they expect it will decrease healthcare costs or improve patient's care and safety. For example, computerization of prescription increases time needed for prescription but could increase patients' safety by providing the information to all healthcare staff involved in a patient's care [16]. Thus, top managers have to choose between these objectives: decreasing time for prescribing and accountability of prescription for patients' safety. Otherwise, without defining operational objectives, this may prove to be wishful thinking, seeing technology as a "magic bullet" to solve diverse and possibly unrelated problems. Thus, "magical thinking" associated with new information technologies results in a tendency to underestimate the risk, effort, and time required. Unrealistic expectations, undermined motivation, scope creep, and wishful thinking have already been identified as risk factors for IT projects by Nelson [17].

Other considerations can also influence top managers and lead them to decisions to adopt a technology: financial incentives by governments or local policy makers and mimicry as the imitation of other organizations' managers' decisions.

3.4 Critical Factors for Telemedicine Implementation

The success of telehealth program, as a viable alternative service delivery or collaboration mode, addresses attention to both technological and managerial issues [7]. Different barriers to the use of telemedicine technology in healthcare organizations have been examined [18, 19] that represent essential factors or issues for implementation of telemedicine technology. Below we briefly review some critical success factor of implementation of telemedicine project.

Broens [20] identified the following factors that influence implementations of telemedicine: (1) technology, (2) acceptance, (3) financing, (4) organization, and (5) policy and legislation.

3.4.1 Technology Issues

Whatever sort of teledentistry system is being designed, several aspects have to be taken into account, related to technical and informational aspects. Fitch et al. [21]

indicate that there are common technological issues that need to be addressed for telemedicine software: reliability and availability, usability, security and confidentiality, efficiency, interoperability, integrability, portability, configurability, and maintainability.

Reliability and availability—The reliability of a system "measures the extent to which the system delivers the service expected of it by its users." Reliability is important because unreliability is usually unpredictable and can cause errors and consequences that might not be immediately obvious to the user [21]. The systematic literature review on electronic health records provided by Boonstra et al. [22] points out the importance of hardware availability and system reliability, in terms of speed and a lack of failures. These issues concern also telemedicine, which may be considered as an interorganizational EHR.

Usability—The usability of a system reflects how easy it is for a user to operate it successfully and to avoid making errors. This issue has been largely investigating in the IS literature [23, 24] and is especially critical in telemedicine [25] and in teledentistry [26, 27].

Security and confidentiality—Security concerns quality of information and includes availability, confidentiality, and integrity of information [21]. This issue is particularly pregnant in teledentistry, highlighting the adequacy of the information obtained via a teleconsultation with a focus on orthodontics and problems concerning the confidentiality of patient records [28].

Efficiency—Efficiency relates to a system's use of resources to perform its task [21]. Teledentistry involves an integration of networking technologies with healthcare processes and often requires applications running on heterogeneous computing environments [21].

Interoperability and integrability—Interoperability is a major issue in information exchange among healthcare professionals [29] and telemedicine [30, 31]. Interoperability and integrability are related to the ease with which one system can operate alongside others [21]. For other authors [31], interoperability is a unique characteristic of healthcare environment. In teledentistry, medical data are useful when shared with medical providers, and it is sometimes difficult due to the sensitive nature of patient records [31]. Telemedicine systems are more prone to this problem than other health IT. Teledentistry is often performed outside the confines of a single organization, and many applications involve cross-discipline and even cross-sector working, while in real-time telemedicine systems, the amount of data transmitted can be very considerable [21]. Video and audio signals have to retain their integrity and arrive at the destination in the state intended by the sender.

Maintainability—Maintainability relates to the ease with which such changes can be made [21]. Romanow et al. specify that health IT performance with respect to interoperability continues to lag other industries, because of the continued use of proprietary systems and databases. As a result, medical data are often locked away in silos of information guarded over by providers outside of the hospital network [31]. Examining how the technological barriers to telemedicine impact telemedicine utilization rates, Paul et al. [18] show a mismatch between the sophistication of the technology and end-user requirements for clinical activities.

Furthermore, support end-user and technical training may be major barriers to telemedicine rate utilization [18] as a prior experience or exposure to computer or health technology [32].

Technical aspects include also the complexity of the existing technology (software and hardware) because it introduces additional problems of systems integration and adequate processing speed and security [33].

Beyond the technical aspect, the quality of the information provided by teledentistry is a key aspect. Boonstra et al. [22] pointed out inadequate recording of patient information and information overload as major problems for the electronic information exchange, which may be extended to telemedicine projects and consequently to teledentistry.

3.4.2 Acceptance Issues

Authors showed that both patients' and professionals' attitudes toward teledentistry technology influence the success of teledentistry implementation. The idea of acceptance is related to perceived usefulness and ease of use [23]. The attitude of medical staff has been found to be a significant determinant of technology adoption in telemedicine innovation implementation [7].

Nurses' acceptance in particular is a crucial factor for the success of teledentistry, and it is connected to their professional roles and status [26]. Oral teleconsultation is a new task for them; in addition to the technology, they have to accept providing this new service. Teledentistry project entails significant changes in nurses' work processes that affect the material conditions of their work and their relationships with other healthcare professionals and their practices [34]. The nurse's acceptance of teledentistry is particularly important; high levels of acceptance can overcome problems with the technology itself and even with a lack of adequate resourcing [35].

The acceptance of patients is also an important issue in teledentistry implementation [26]. Therefore, Giraudeau et al. [36] identify lack of trust on the side of patients, in France, and Patel and Antonarakis [28] quote concerns about the lack of direct patient contact, in the UK, as a problematic acceptance issue.

3.4.3 Financing Issues

According to Broens et al. [20], financing issues are important especially when implementation of teledentistry is widespread. Other authors have highlighted the importance of a feasible business model for telemedicine [37]. The implementation of teledentistry influences the financial situation of various stakeholders in the healthcare process and leads to a redistribution of costs and revenues which is different to the financing of traditional (i.e., non-telemedicine) dental care. In France, there are various legal and ethical constraints that prevent the establishment of a viable business model for teledentistry including the reluctance of health insurance companies to pay for acts of telemedicine [36, 38]. In the longer term, this will inevitably involve changes to and reform of the current legal framework that governs telemedicine.

3.4.4 Organizational Issues

Telemedicine implementation concerns also organizational issues. The resistance to health IT (HIT) and especially physician's resistance to HIT are contextual characteristics of healthcare environment [31, 39–41]. The cause of this resistance can be traced by the manner in which physicians work and control their work, independent of hierarchical control and relied on collegial control [31] and professional autonomy, related to high skills required to handle complex work [42]. Nevertheless, as Berg assumes, "whether an information system is successful or not is decided on the workplace" [43]; consequently, teledentistry has to deal with this professional autonomy in order to prevent resistance. In addition, the implementation and use of teledentistry technology, as an innovation, affect the boundaries of healthcare organizations and require new external collaborations with other healthcare organizations.

IT implementations are known to cause significant changes in employees' job characteristics [44].

Authors investigate also how technology-triggered change processes and identified evident changes in skills and tasks triggered by implementation of the IT system in health organization, for physicians, nurses, and ancillary staff [45].

A big concern is the new relationship between the clinical telehealth providers and the information technology (IT) providers that are needed to implement the tools used for the consultation and diagnosis by dentists [26, 35].

Implementing teledentistry projects requires strong managerial support and champions who are able to find a compromise among the stakeholders [46, 47]. Previous research [48] has identified ten different types of adopters in telehealth projects: enthusiastic user, positive user, critical user, hesitant user, positive participant, hesitant participant, critical participant, neutral participant, negative participant, and positive nonparticipant. This issue fits acceptance concerns and the questions of the resistance of healthcare professionals.

Moreover, recent studies on electronic medical records highlighted several problems as inadequate training, insufficient support for change, lack of user involvement, lack of recognition by the top management of the key actors, the workload during the implementation phase and of the concertation of the actors, the lack of time dedicated to user training, the failure strategic alignment between the administration and the main medical leaders, the lack of effective internal communication strategy, and the lack of anticipation of technological risks (business interruption, failure) [49].

Dealing with all these aspects needs a project management approach, as a main factor for a successful implementation. Nelson [17] identified and prioritized the risk factors for all IT projects. Lack of project champion, project ambiguity, lack of required knowledge or skills, changes to membership on the project team, and insufficient resources are considered as main risk factors associated with projects of implementation of clinical information systems [17], which can be extended to telemedicine and teledentistry projects.

Moreover, telemedicine has to deal with different stakeholders involved as governments, healthcare providers, general practitioners, and patients in a multidisciplinary and cooperative context, implying different goals [15].

3.4.5 Policy and Legislation Issues

Teledentistry raises numerous questions such as the issues related to the transfer of medical data, the definition of acts of teledentistry, and the legal limits on cost sharing and payment between different medical specialties. Privacy concerns about digital patient records and medical data are examples of core contextual variables in health information technology [31] and are a recurrent theme in HIT literature [31, 50, 51].

Different authors [18, 22, 29] showed that patient confidentiality and privacy issues are impacting HIT and telemedicine.

In the longer term, social policy and legislation issues will be crucial to the economic viability of teledentistry.

Conclusion

Technology, acceptance, organization, policy, and legislation have to be identified and apprehended in order to move from pilot phase to successfully large-scale teledentistry. These issues have been assessed for projects in the information systems field, but they are more crucial in health sector for telemedicine projects because of the autonomy of the healthcare professionals and the potential effects of technology breakdowns and errors in the information chain on medical errors and the effectiveness of patients' care. Paradoxically, top managers, decision-makers, and sponsors could be tempted to underestimate the importance of this analysis and, globally, of the change management involving all the stakeholders because of the time and money needed. Nevertheless, they have to consider this part as an investment, not a cost, in order to achieve expected benefits.

References

1. Bradley M, Black P, Noble S, Thompson R, Lamey PJ. Application of teledentistry in oral medicine in a community dental service, N. Ireland. Br Dent J. 2010;209:399–404. https://doi.org/10.1038/sj.bdj.2010.928.
2. Golder DT, Brennan KA. Practicing dentistry in the age of telemedicine. J Am Dent Assoc. 2000;1939(131):734–44.
3. Jampani ND, Nutalapati R, Dontula BSK, Boyapati R. Applications of teledentistry: a literature review and update. J Int Soc Prev Community Dent. 2011;1:37–44. https://doi.org/10.4103/2231-0762.97695.

4. Scuffham PA, Steed M. An economic evaluation of the Highlands and Islands teledentistry project. J Telemed Telecare. 2002;8:165–77. https://doi.org/10.1258/135763302320118915.
5. Bhambal A, Saxena S, Balsaraf SV. Teledentistry: potentials unexplored! J Int Oral Health. 2010;2:1–6.
6. Sanchez Dils E, Lefebvre C, Abeyta K. Teledentistry in the United States: a new horizon of dental care. Int J Dent Hyg. 2004;2:161–4. https://doi.org/10.1111/j.1601-5037.2004.00093.x.
7. Hu PJ-H, Chau PYK, Sheng ORL. Adoption of telemedicine technology by healthcare organizations: an exploratory study. J Organ Comput Electron Commer. 2002;12:197–221. https://doi.org/10.1207/S15327744JOCE1203_01.
8. Mariño R, Ghanim A. Teledentistry: a systematic review of the literature. J Telemed Telecare. 2013;19:179–83. https://doi.org/10.1177/1357633X13479704.
9. Jackson DE, McClean SI. Trends in telemedicine assessment indicate neglect of key criteria for predicting success. J Health Organ Manag. 2012;26:508–23.
10. Hu PH, Chau PY, Chan YK, Kwok JCK. Investigating technology implementation in a neurosurgical teleconsultation program: a case study in Hong Kong. In: proceedings of the 34th annual Hawaii international conference on system sciences. Washington, DC: IEEE; 2001. p. 9pp.
11. EHTEL. Sustainable telemedicine: paradigms for future-proof healthcare—eHealth Portal for Europe [WWW Document]. 2008. URL https://www.ehtel.eu/references-files/tf-cdm-telemedicine/ehtel-briefing-paper-sustainable-telemedicine-paradigms-for-future-proof-healthcare. Accessed 28 Apr 16.
12. Ekeland AG, Grøttland A. Assessment of MAST in European patient-centered telemedicine pilots. Int J Technol Assess Health Care. 2015;31:304–11. https://doi.org/10.1017/S0266462315000574.
13. Kidholm K, Ekeland AG, Jensen LK, Rasmussen J, Pedersen CD, Bowes A, Flottorp SA, Bech M. A model for assessment of telemedicine applications: MAST. Int J Technol Assess Health Care. 2012;28:44–51. https://doi.org/10.1017/S0266462311000638.
14. Ekeland AG, Bowes A, Flottorp S. Effectiveness of telemedicine: a systematic review of reviews. Int J Med Inform. 2010;79(11):736–71. https://doi.org/10.1016/j.ijmed- inf.2010.08.006 20.
15. Masella C, Zanaboni P. Assessment models for telemedicine services in National Health Systems. Int J Healthc Technol Manag. 2008;9:446–72. https://doi.org/10.1504/IJHTM.2008.020198.
16. Hollingworth W, Devine EB, Hansen RN, Lawless NM, Comstock BA, Wilson-Norton JL, Tharp KL, Sullivan SL. The impact of e-prescribing on prescriber and staff time in ambulatory care clinics: a time–motion study. J Am Med Inform Assoc. 2007;14(6):722–30. https://doi.org/10.1197/jamia.M2377.
17. Nelson RR. IT project management: infamous failures, classic mistakes, and best practices. MIS Q Exec. 2007;6(2):67–78.
18. Paul DL, Pearlson KE, McDaniel RR. Assessing technological barriers to telemedicine: technology-management implications. IEEE Trans Eng Manag. 1999;46:279–88. https://doi.org/10.1109/17.775280.
19. Tanriverdi H, Iacono CS. Diffusion of telemedicine: a knowledge barrier perspective. Telemed J. 1999;5:223–44. https://doi.org/10.1089/107830299311989.
20. Broens THF, in't Veld RMHAH, Vollenbroek-Hutten MMR, Hermens HJ, van Halteren AT, Nieuwenhuis LJM. Determinants of successful telemedicine implementations: a literature study. J Telemed Telecare. 2007;13:303–9. https://doi.org/10.1258/135763307781644951.
21. Fitch CJ, Briggs JS, Beresford RA. System issues for successful tele-medicine implementation. Health Informatics J. 2000;6:166–73. https://doi.org/10.1177/146045820000600310.
22. Boonstra A, Versluis A, Vos JF. Implementing electronic health records in hospitals: a systematic literature review. BMC Health Serv Res. 2014;14(1):370. https://doi.org/10.1186/1472-6963-14-370.
23. Davis FD, Bagozzi RP, Warshaw PR. User acceptance of computer technology: a comparison of two theoretical models. Manag Sci. 1989;35:982.
24. Venkatesh V, Morris MG, Davis GB, Davis FD. User acceptance of information technology: toward a unified view. MIS Q. 2003;27:425–78.

25. Chau PYK, Hu PJ-H. Investigating healthcare professionals' decisions to accept telemedicine technology: an empirical test of competing theories. Inf Manag. 2002;39:297–311. https://doi.org/10.1016/S0378-7206(01)00098-2.
26. Petcu R, Ologeanu-Taddei R, Bourdon I, Kimble C, Giraudeau N. Acceptance and organizational aspects of oral tele-consultation: a French STUDY. In: 2016 49th Hawaii International Conference on System Sciences (HICSS). IEEE; 2016. p. 3124–3132. https://doi.org/10.1109/HICSS.2016.393.
27. Whitten PS, Richardson JD. A scientific approach to the assessment of telemedicine acceptance. J Telemed Telecare. 2002;8:246–8. https://doi.org/10.1258/135763302320272257.
28. Patel RN, Antonarakis GS. Factors influencing the adoption and implementation of teledentistry in the UK, with a focus on orthodontics. Community Dent Oral Epidemiol. 2013;41:424–31. https://doi.org/10.1111/cdoe.12029.
29. Zwaanswijk M, Verheij RA, Wiesman FJ, Friele RD. Benefits and problems of electronic information exchange as perceived by health care professionals: an interview study. BMC Health Serv Res. 2011;11(1):256.
30. Ganguly P, Ray P. Software interoperability of telemedicine systems: a CSCW perspective. In: seventh international conference on parallel and distributed systems, 2000. Proceedings. Los Alamitos: IEEE; 2000. p. 349–356. doi:https://doi.org/10.1109/ICPADS.2000.857717.
31. Romanow D, Cho S, Straub D. Riding the wave: past trends and future directions for health IT research. MIS Q. 2012;36:iii–A18.
32. Or CK, Karsh BT. A systematic review of patient acceptance of consumer health information technology. J Am Med Inform Assoc. 2009;16(4):550–60.
33. Barki H, Rivard S, Talbot J. Toward an assessment of software development risk. J Manag Inf Syst. 1993;10(2):203–25.
34. Nicolini D. The work to make telemedicine work: a social and articulative view. Soc Sci Med. 2006;62:2754–67. https://doi.org/10.1016/j.socscimed.2005.11.001.
35. Wade VA, Eliott JA, Hiller JE. Clinician acceptance is the key factor for sustainable telehealth services. Qual Health Res. 2014;24:682–94. https://doi.org/10.1177/1049732314528809.
36. Giraudeau N, Valcarcel J, Tassery H, Levallois B, Cuisinier F, Tramini P, Vialla F. Projet e-DENT : téléconsultation bucco-dentaire en EHPAD. Eur Res Telemed. 2015;3:51. https://doi.org/10.1016/j.eurtel.2014.04.005.
37. Chen S, Cheng A, Mehta K. A review of telemedicine business models. Telemed e-Health. 2013;19(4):287–97.
38. Ologeanu-Taddei R, Bourdon I, Kimble C, Giraudeau N. The acceptability of teleconsultations in teledentistry: a case study. In: Cruz-Cunha M, Miranda I, editors. Encyclopedia of e-health and telemedicine. Hershey: IGI Global; 2016. p. 1–12. https://doi.org/10.4018/978-1-4666-9978-6.ch072.
39. Bhattacherjee A, Hikmet N. Physicians' resistance toward healthcare information technology: a theoretical model and empirical test. Eur J Inf Syst. 2007;16:725–37. https://doi.org/10.1057/palgrave.ejis.3000717.
40. Lapointe L, Rivard S. Getting physicians to accept new information technology: insights from case studies. Can Med Assoc J. 2006;174:1573–8. https://doi.org/10.1503/cmaj.050281.
41. Lapointe L, Rivard S. A multilevel model of resistance to information technology implementation. MIS Q. 2005;29:461–91.
42. Mintzberg H. The structuring of organization: a synthesis of the research. Englewood Cliffs: Prentice-Hall; 1990.
43. Berg M. Implementing information systems in health care organizations: myths and challenges. International Journal of Medical Informatics. 2001;64(2):143–56.
44. Bala H, Venkatesh V. Changes in employees' job characteristics during an enterprise system implementation: a latent growth modeling perspective. MIS Q. 2013;37:1113–A7.
45. Davidson EJ, Chismar WG. The interaction of institutionally triggered and technology-triggered social structure change: an investigation of computerized physician order entry. MIS Q. 2007;31:739–58.
46. Wade V, Eliott J. The role of the champion in telehealth service development: a qualitative analysis. J Telemed Telecare. 2012;18:490–2. https://doi.org/10.1258/jtt.2012.GTH115.

47. Wade VA, Hamlyn JS. The relationship between telehealth and information technology ranges from that of uneasy bedfellows to creative partnerships. J Telemed Telecare. 2013;19:401–4. https://doi.org/10.1177/1357633X13506533.
48. Vuononvirta T, Timonen M, Keinänen-Kiukaanniemi S, Timonen O, Ylitalo K, Kanste O, Taanila A. The attitudes of multiprofessional teams to telehealth adoption in northern Finland health centres. J Telemed Telecare. 2009;15(6):290–6. https://doi.org/10.1258/jtt.2009.090108.
49. Cresswell K, Sheikh A. Organizational issues in the implementation and adoption of health information technology innovations: an interpretative review. International Journal of Medical Informatics. 2013;82(5):e73–e86.
50. Anderson CL, Agarwal R. The digitization of healthcare: boundary risks, emotion, and consumer willingness to disclose personal health information. Inf Syst Res. 2011;22:469–90. https://doi.org/10.1287/isre.1100.0335.
51. Angst CM, Agarwal R. Adoption of electronic health records in the presence of privacy concerns: the elaboration likelihood model and individual persuasion. MIS Q. 2009;33:339–70.

Ethics and Teledentistry: Challenges and Questions

4

Olivier Hamel

Abstract
Think about practice and its ethical issues.

Keywords
Dentistry • Ethics • Telemedicine

4.1 Introduction

Naturally, when one thinks of "telemedicine", where the health worker is physically absent, one perceives a profound transformation of the most important facet of medicine: the patient/practitioner relationship.

To reflect on the ethical nature of this subject fundamentally boils down to asking one's self about the impact that this recent practice has on the very particular interpersonal relationship, that is, the relationship of health care, at the time of a consultation. It consists of balancing the practice of telemedicine with protecting the person undergoing the dental tele-consultation.

As far as the authors of this paper are aware, no research in medical ethics currently exists, which specifically examines telemedicine in dentistry.

O. Hamel
Faculty of Dental Surgery, Université Paul Sabatier Toulouse 3
[Paul Sabatier University, Toulouse 3], Toulouse, France

Medical and Biological Ethics Laboratory, EA 4569, Faculty of Medicine,
Paris Descartes University, Paris, France
e-mail: olivier.hamel@univ-tlse3.fr

N. Giraudeau (ed.), *e-Health Care in Dentistry and Oral Medicine*,
https://doi.org/10.1007/978-3-319-69450-4_4

This paper will therefore attempt to imagine the issues that may serve as the basis for such research. In light of the development of the practice, it can be predicted that said research will soon become pertinent and legitimate.

An attempt will also be made herein to outline how social and psychological aspects are just as serious as the reliability of the systems.

After briefly introducing some texts, which are designed to regulate these practices, six ethical issues will be described.

4.2 International Ethical Framework [1]

The *Universal Declaration of Human Rights* (United Nations, 1948) is a legally binding instrument on an international level of which Article 12 is dedicated to privacy protection. The International Court of Justice, which was founded in order to resolve disputes between nations within the framework of this declaration, has given no ruling that is particularly pertinent as to how to interpret this text. Nevertheless, it is cited before national courts within the context of privacy disputes.

The World Medical Association (WMA) International Code of Medical Ethics (1949, amended version of 2006) stipulates that doctors must respect the patient's right to confidentiality; "It is ethical to disclose confidential information when there is a real imminent threat of harm to the patient or to others and this threat can only be removed by a breach of confidentiality".

The WMA's Declaration on Medical Ethics and Advanced Medical Technology (2002) outlines that the patient's safety must be fully taken into account when developing and applying medical technologies.

In the WMA's Declaration of Lisbon on the Rights of the Patient (1981, amended version of 2005), the WMA raises professional secrecy, a guarantor of confidentiality, but also the right to quality care. The Declaration outlines the obligation of the doctor to cooperate with other health-care providers treating the patient to coordinate medical prescriptions. Confidentiality covers the following fields:

a. All identifiable information about a patient's health status, medical condition, diagnosis and treatment and all other information of a personal kind must be kept confidential, even after death. Exceptionally, the descendant may have a right of access to information that would inform them of their health risks.
b. Confidential information can only be disclosed if the patient gives explicit consent or expressly provided for in the law. Information can be disclosed to other health care providers only on a strict "need to know" basis unless the patient has given explicit consent.
c. All identifiable patient data must be protected. The protection of the data must be appropriate to the manner of its storage. Human substances from which identifiable data can be derived must be likewise protected.

   (World Medical Association: *Declaration of Lisbon on the Rights of the Patient*, 1981, amended version 2005)

The cited texts refer to medicine, and it is clear that they neither directly target nor concern dental surgery, which is not to say that one should not reflect upon it.

4.3 What Are the Ethical Issues in Dentistry with Regard to Telemedicine?

4.3.1 Telemedicine's Place Within Health Care

Technology is becoming more and more of a constant fixture every day, and it is possible to imagine a new skill set for those dealing with dental matters: dental surgeons, of course, but also nurses, nurses' aids, dental assistants, etc. They could become "e-health-care providers"—this may even be the emergence of a new profession.

And these health-care providers would be even more commonplace in a sector where they have already been multiplying for decades. Furthermore, various professionals are already brought together to collaborate in caring for one patient: biologists, radiologists, orthodontists, implantologists, periodontists and, of course, general practitioners [2]. The data contained within the file is thus shared.

Confronted as they are today with difficulties accessing health care that are often linked to a demanding professional demography, e-health-care provider(s) would be able to respond to patients' needs. A nurse's aid who is trained to perform this technique and care can, with a dental surgeon in remote space and time, play an essential role in the dental care plan of an elderly person living in a nursing home.

In this example, the dental surgeon's remoteness obliges the nurse's aid to undertake relationships with the patient almost entirely on his or her own. Beyond having the technical ability, it seems necessary for the nurse's aid to be sensitised to certain aspects specific to health-care relationships when they concern teeth and dental cavities. If the nurse's aid, who is nevertheless used to often having frequent bodily intimacy with the patient, were to have an understanding of the symbolic value that the mouth and teeth have, from the perspective of pleasure, satiety and even desire, this would help them to acknowledge that even placing an intra-oral camera in a patient's mouth represents more than just an innocuous action.

There would be a twofold benefit to using medical psychology or psycho-dentistry to acquire this skill: for both the nurse's aid, who would be able to perform this exercise calmly (and it is known how nurse's aids often encounter and describe hesitations when dealing with dental care), and for the patient, who would have a trained and engaged health-care provider as an intermediary.

In more general terms, in light of this increase in technical know-how and the observation that health-care providers are multiplying, this is imagined to be an opportunity for dental professionals to become involved. The dream is the following quasi-ideal situation: the role of the dental surgeon becoming or having the ability to become central and considered to be a fully fledged player in health care and customised medical and/or dental records enabling different health-care providers to coordinate on the core component, the patient.

4.3.2 Prevention: A Major Ethical Issue

Far too often, the culture of care still takes precedence over the culture of prevention, at least in France. Therefore, the following question is posed: does prevention really represent a major ethical issue, as the authors believe it does, for all medical partners?

Developing telemedicine in dentistry could become an exceptional opportunity for collaboration between different medical players. The evolution of the profession, the role of therapeutic education [3] and the possible creation of a new vocation within oral health and "hygienists" are all recurring themes which call our values into question. Hygienists, being paramedic staff who are mainly focused on prevention and who are already present in many countries, would be able to make full use of this "telemedicine" tool in order to initiate preventative actions. The potential population is just as a varied as the possible age groups, concerned by both preventing individual instances of decay and that of gum disease.

4.3.3 The Patient's Freedom of Choice

Within health-care institutions, unless the patient opposes, they are presumed to consent to their data being both exchanged and shared by the "care team". Whether in their house, their residency or a surrogate home, such as residential Care Homes for the Elderly, health-care professionals can exchange information regarding the person whom they ensure to care for and follow up on, with each other. Once the data has been recorded in a database, the patient must give their express consent for the data to be shared and each time that any health-care professional accesses it. The same applies in pooling structures, such as multi-professional care homes.

The advent of digital technology within health care can sometimes fuel fears relating to disclosing information of a private nature or the dehumanising of the relationship between the caregiver and the care receiver. And yet, it must be acknowledged that information and communication technologies can enable beneficial circulation of pertinent information for the continuity of care, while cyber security and access controls reinforce the protection of citizens' personal data [4].

The classic example discussed previously shall be returned to here: a patient in a Care Home for the Elderly needs to undergo a consultation in "e-health" mode. The nurse will carry out the tele-consultation using an intra-oral camera. A few days later, the dental surgeon, or perhaps one should say "a" dental surgeon, will give his or her report and suggest a care plan.

Who is then at the centre of this famous "unusual consultation" who links the patient with the practitioner? The nurse seems to play this role; however, the nurse lacks the ability to respond to any questions the patient may ask about his or her dental or gingival pain. Does the "remote" dentist not become a simple service provider, and to what extent is the patient or are his or her relatives free to choose the person, now the "oral cavity technician", who will be able to know their state and issue advice, wherein lies the so-described relationship of trust to validate a caregiver/care receiver relationship, in accordance with the current perceptions on information and consent?

This is exactly where the word "consent" resonates in the sense that "the patient consents!" And, rather than to consent, the authors hold that the verb "to choose" is no doubt more gratifying for each of the counterparts, both patient and practitioner.

It can be affirmed that the relationship of trust is vital, even if the practitioner is not directly present. Technology must not cloud the fact that it is still a human being there, awaiting skill and understanding.

Could tacit consent, rather than choice, be accepted when it is guided by considerations particular to the organisation of the team in charge of making the tele-diagnosis?

In France today, dental tele-consultations are still only offered on a small scale and tend to be mainly a public provision relayed by housing institutes. What would happen if this provision became a private enterprise? The quasi-spontaneous trust in the hospital institution gives comfort to the principle held that a patient who grants this trust accepts for an unidentified caregiver to assume responsibility for them.

But how about if tele-dentistry were to become a market, an e-business? How could the patient be free to choose or refuse any service being provided when it is heavily promoted?

The individual responsibility of each health-care provider must be integrated, so that information and communication technologies continue to be used at the sole benefit of the patient [5].

4.3.4 Protecting the Person

Another matter to be considered is the confidentiality of a consultation, whatever the technology being used is. Within the context of remote medicine, machines seem to render the problem more complex.

There are two situations which should probably be differentiated here, depending on whether telemedicine is used in an emergency or not. It seems easier to maintain confidentiality in the instance of remote dentistry, at least whenever the consultation is not carried out in a state of emergency. The risk of disclosing any aspect of one's private life, or even simply a face, is much greater in a consultation that is carried out in a more direct and urgent context. However, it must be admitted that this seems to be restricted to a few very particular tele-consultation cases, such as for people out at sea, for instance, or, even more rarely, for people in space.

In a more everyday instance, video conferences ultimately become the common base for many telemedicine applications. Respecting ethics therefore seems like a fairly simple matter and one which concerns the questions of data security and respecting medical secrecy. However, this complexity is not as new as it may seem, and these questions about the security of storing medical information and data have already been raised since IT arrived in dental surgeries a few decades ago. It shall therefore be seen that this line of questioning is perhaps not the most essential one.

In any case, the sick person, being the object or subject of telemedicine, must be protected by the scientist, the lawmaker and the lawyer, who are all united by an approach that is guided by ethics. Should an additional normative context be conceived? Probably not if the legal framework of the care relationship has already been installed: indeed, should it be different?

To just mention something, which is of major importance: what happens if a serious disease is unexpectedly discovered during the course of a tele-consultation? The reality of the practice then goes beyond regulatory aspects.

4.3.5 Assessment and Research in Telemedicine

Telemedicine and especially tele-dentistry have not been around for long. For this reason, the knowledge of its impact, its efficiency and the perspectives on it are still limited. No medical discipline can ethically forgo an assessment based on valid scientific research: research on telemedicine (Which new technical devices are they and how effective are they? What are the advantages, etc.?) but also research into the ethics of this subject (What are the issues that exist with the practice?). As ethics and money are closely related, the ethical aspects of these new expenditures to be envisaged need to be dealt with from the perspective of both individual and collective benefit.

When the economic, social and legal aspects are assessed, there should also be an assessment of the users' professionalism and skills. Recognising the skills and qualifications induced from using telemedicine applications must be accompanied by treatments being codified and, thus, health-care facilitators being paid fairly.

4.3.6 A Public Health Social Challenge

How legitimate is tele-dentistry? Its feasibility will depend on public health in the broad sense of the term and the reality of health-care professionals' actions.

Will tele-dentistry be an additional opportunity for dentists to be considered public health clinicians and to take full responsibility?

To take responsibility consists of asking one's self about the notion of fair care, about that of the place and role of institutions in regulating practices while considering prevention to be a major issue.

There is no doubt that it is too early to make any claims about the role that tele-dentistry has in the provision of access to health care. However, insofar as tele-consultations have the ability to encompass various vulnerabilities (age, handicaps, etc.), it can already be affirmed that by bringing this additional benefit to care, dental tele-consultations can constitute a real ethical challenge.

4.4 Discussion/Conclusion

Whether they are direct or indirect, consultations are an essential part of medical care [6]. A consultation is like the reflection of the patient's life. Consultations expose a person's state of health and bear witness to his or her degree of vulnerability. The subtle intersubjective relationship which is then created between the caregiver and the care receiver requires listening, caution and respect. Christian Hervé describes a series of ruptures, which objectify this vulnerability. The rupture of self-worth explains the inability to mobilise one's strengths to organise their care. Then, the rupture of usual time references means that one's whole life revolves around the sickness and conversations about physical and/or intellectual limitations. In time, the patient will need to fashion a new reality about what his or her body or intellect can henceforth undertake.

With regard to these ruptures, Paul Ricoeur [7] translated the loss of self-worth, as the fact of no longer being an actor in one's own life, of becoming particularly passive in one's own life and of no longer having freedom and autonomy. It is therefore the caregiver's duty to maintain a relationship, which combines probity and responsibility. Thus, access to freedom and greater autonomy arises from the caregiver/care receiver relationship, such as equity which occurs through accessing care guaranteed by a health-care pledge established; thus, the pledge is characterised by the three fundamental notions of respecting medical confidentiality, the right to the truth, and obtaining enlightened consent.

What place does telemedicine have within this objective? What are the secrets for protecting this nature of consultation, if not that of interpersonal and comprehensive communication?

Research work on narrative medicine [8] has shown that in medicine, the patient's listening time is limited to 18 s. Do tele-consultations enable this to go further? This is not at all certain.

The act of existing needs to be rethought, from the patient's perspective. The overriding objective of consultations must be to mobilise and develop the mentalities of the public, the patients' loved ones, professional or family carers and even those of the patients.

So, admittedly, there are more and more computing means (like telemedicine) which are aimed at creating a link between hospital health-care professionals and those in town, to ensure that follow-up is effective in terms of quality of care but also in terms of efficiency. French law, in particular [9], promotes the multiprofessional aspect of facilitators: this is particularly useful in terms of efficiency for providing optimal care to patients affected by chronic diseases, who are often elderly and are losing their autonomy or are perhaps dependent and handicapped and always vulnerable. With regard to information being exchanged, in terms of words, as well as gestures or behaviour, discernment is to be encouraged. In this way, what is exchanged are not secrets, but rather information deemed to be indispensable for a colleague to know at a given moment so that these decisions ensure optimal benefits to the patient (or the least possible damage) and that of collectivity in terms of well-managed resources.

Rather than protecting data, it is privacy and the repercussions of the illness which matter.

Telemedicine is perhaps more than an additional tool for medical or dental practice. It is a different way of organising health care, which aims to put the patient at the centre of the health system, in contrast to institutional, state or corporate approaches.

In France today, it seems that all conditions, which would lead to telemedicine and tele-health platforms being deployed coherently on a national level, are fulfilled [10]:

- From the perspective of patients and users: needs are clearly expressed. Telemedicine and tele-health platforms constitute tools which help in responding to the new challenges brought by the ageing of the population and the medical exodus from rural or isolated areas, as well as performing everyday medicine.

- From the perspective of health-care professionals: guaranteed training and especially guaranteed close support and help with the changeover to using "Information and Communication Health technology" tools which are not necessarily intuitive to use.
- From the perspective of ethics and responsibility: guaranteed confidentiality and interoperability, in conformity with the regulations.
- From the perspective of industrial deployment and employment: telemedicine and tele-health procedures enable new employment opportunities to be envisaged so that the services can be provided on a regional level.

This reflection is ever the more necessary in the face of technological advances. Ethical reflections on both the legitimacy of sharing information and also the possible consequences are part of accountability ethics, which are only capable of protecting patients against inopportune disclosure.

In conclusion, while sharing data is a big deal, protecting a person's privacy is the objective.

References

1. Ferraud-Ciandet N. Ethique et droit de la télémédecine en Argentine. In: Les systèmes informatisés complexes en santé. Banque de données, télémédecine: normes et enjeux éthiques. Paris: Dalloz; 2013. p. 21–34.
2. Denost H, Blaizot A, Trentesaux T, Hamel O. Médecine bucco-dentaire et valeurs éthiques: quelles spécificités. Ethics Med Public Health. 2016;2:181–5.
3. Trentesaux T, Delfosse C, Ternois M, Rousset M-M, Hervé C, Hamel O. L'éducation thérapeutique du patient, un concept applicable en odontologie pédiatrique? Rev Francophone d'Odontol Pédiatrique. 2009;4:52–6.
4. Lucas J. Le partage des données personnelles de santé dans les usages du numérique en santé à l'épreuve du consentement exprès de la personne. In: Les systèmes informatisés complexes en santé. Banque de données, télémédecine : normes et enjeux éthiques. Paris: Dalloz; 2013. p. 39–56.
5. Déclaration du Conseil Européen des Ordres des Médecins sur la télémédecine. Bari. 2014. Disponible sur https://www.conseil-national.medecin.fr/.
6. Hervé C, Mamzer M-F. La consultation médicale à l'épreuve d'une nouvelle humanisation: quelle évolution éthique pour le médecin et son patient? Ethics Med Public Health. 2016;2:238–45.
7. Ricoeur P. Soi-même comme un autre. Paris: Ed Le Seuil; 1990.
8. Charon R. Narrative and medicine. N Engl J Med. 2004;350(9):862–4.
9. Loi du 4 mars 2002 relative aux droits des malades et à la qualité du système de santé. Disponible sur https://www.legifrance.gouv.fr/.
10. Pavageau E. Rôle de l'industriel en tant qu'opérateur technique de service "e-santé", pour le professionnel de santé et pour l'usager. In: Les systèmes informatisés complexes en santé. Banque de données, télémédecine: normes et enjeux éthiques. Paris: Dalloz; 2013. p. 95–120.

The Economics of Teledentistry

5

Gregoire Mercier and Rodrigo Jose Marino

Abstract

Teledentistry has the potential to improve health system performance in terms of efficiency and equity. Efficiency can be assessed either alongside a clinical trial or through modeling methods. However the evidence regarding the economic evaluations of teledentistry programs is scarce. Methodological guidelines dedicated to the economic evaluation of teledentistry might help researcher to design and implement such evaluations.

Keywords

Teledentistry • Efficiency • Economic evaluation • Equity

5.1 Introduction: Efficiency Is a Key Dimension of Health System Performance

Teledentistry (TD) is the use of information technology and telecommunications for dental care, consultation and education. TD has the potential to improve health system performance.

G. Mercier (✉)
Department of Medical Information, Montpellier University Hospital, Montpellier, France
e-mail: g-mercier@chu-montpellier.fr

R.J. Marino
Oral Health Cooperative Research Centre, Melbourne Dental School, University of Melbourne, Melbourne, VIC, Australia
e-mail: r.marino@unimelb.edu.au

N. Giraudeau (ed.), *e-Health Care in Dentistry and Oral Medicine*,
https://doi.org/10.1007/978-3-319-69450-4_5

Assessing the performance of a health system requires a clear definition of its boundaries, as well as an elicitation of the key objectives pursued.

The World Health Organization's definition is 'The resources, actors and institutions related to the financing, regulation and provision of activities which primary intent is to improve or maintain health'. However, other institutions and organizations have proposed other definitions, ranging from narrower boundaries centred on medical care (e.g. OECD) to much wider ones, encompassing all determinants of health including individual behavioural aspects.

Each definition of the health-care system entails different stakeholders whose information needs, communication strategies and goals might not necessarily be aligned. Health system stakeholders include service users, professionals, purchaser organizations, regulators, the government (national or local), researchers and the broader public.

Additionally, each definition refers to a particular set of outcome measures to be included in the assessment. Typically, the five key domains of health-care system performance are population health, health status (clinical quality and appropriateness), responsiveness (including satisfaction and expectations), equity (of access and of finance) and efficiency [1]. Health system performance is multidimensional per se, whatever the boundaries acknowledged.

Teledentistry might lead to better oral health outcomes, to reduce potentially avoidable hospitalizations, to save health-care costs (i.e. efficiency) and to improve access to dental care (i.e. equity). The economic approach to teledentistry focuses on the efficiency component of performance. As such, it is of high importance to all stakeholders. Patients are expecting better dental care, policymakers are willing to foster an intervention aimed to improve outcomes, public and private payers are interested in the efficiency for pricing considerations, and the industry is looking for innovative business models.

Robust data is required by policymakers but findings regarding teledentistry are mixed [2].

In the following sections, we are going to propose a theoretical framework and practical approaches to the assessment of the efficiency of teledentistry. Then, we will briefly review the available published evidence and discuss the opportunity to design methodological guidelines dedicated to the economic evaluation of teledentistry.

5.2 Assessing the Efficiency of Telemedicine: A Theoretical Framework

5.2.1 Efficiency

Efficiency is an increasingly important dimension of health system performance. Efficiency data is useful to a large range of stakeholders: government, regulators, payers and the public. Policymakers are interested in various concepts:

- *Productivity* is the ratio of *outputs* (e.g. physical quantities of episodes of dental care) to inputs (e.g. all resources dedicated to dental care such as facilities, medical and nonmedical staff, equipment, disposables and drugs).

– *Efficiency* is the ratio of *outcomes* (value or quality, e.g. oral health improvement at the population level) to inputs.

The technical efficiency pertains to maximizing outcomes for a given set of inputs (i.e. close to the production possibility frontier), while the allocative efficiency aims to reaching a socially ideal mix of outcomes for a given set of inputs (i.e. close to the social welfare function).

At the macro level, budget allocation is a possible lever to improve efficiency, provided that policymakers are able to identify high-value interventions. The need of decision-making for budget allocation in health care has led to the development of different economic analyses aiming to support decision-making under conditions of uncertainty. Economic evaluation can be defined as the comparative analysis of alternative health-care programmes in terms of their costs and consequences [3]. Economic evaluations are context specific [4] and are useful to the decision-makers when performed and reported accurately [5].

5.2.2 Definitions, Advantages and Disadvantages of the Three Forms of Economic Evaluation

The three forms of comparative economic evaluations that consider both costs and consequences are presented in the following table.

Decision analysis	Consequences	Unit of measurement
Cost-effectiveness analysis (CEA)	Quality **or** quantity of life	Physical units, e.g. oral health score
Cost-utility analysis (CUA)	Quality and quantity of life	QALYs
Cost-benefit analysis (CBA)	Quality and quantity of life	Money, e.g. human capital, willingness to pay

- *CEA* compares costs and effectiveness of treatment alternatives, e.g. teledentistry versus conventional dental care. The effectiveness is a common measure, ideally 'life years gained' as a final outcome. Intermediate outcomes can also be used if the link to the final outcome of importance is established; examples are oral health scores.

Advantages	Disadvantages
Relatively simple to undertake	Single, programme-specific output: other potentially important outcomes may be ignored (e.g. 'life years saved' do not consider morbidity)
	Unidimensionality may result in drawing erroneous conclusions

- *CUA* has its own strengths and limitations. Typical outcome measures are quality-adjusted life years (QALYs), which assume that the only potential benefit from health care is improvement in health-related quality of life. QALYs are overall measures of health outcome that weight the life expectancy of a patient with an estimate of their health-related quality-of-life (utility) score (measured on a 0–1 scale).

Advantages	Disadvantages
CUA measures more aspects of health and well-being than a single natural unit: single or multiple, generic output and the notion of value are incorporated	CUA is more complex to undertake than CEA
Only final effectiveness outcomes (e.g. live years saved) are used, intermediate outputs (e.g. cases found) are unsuitable	The different methods available to estimate QALYs may not provide identical results
CUA recognizes that health treatments and programmes impact upon both length and quality of life and do incorporate weightings of the components	
CUAs are comparable whereas CEA are programme specific	

- *CBA* is the only form of evaluation that addresses the net social benefit of an intervention. It is less commonly used in practice due to the difficulties to express utilities in monetary terms.

Advantages	Disadvantages
Defines whether the benefits of an intervention exceed its costs	CBA can be very complex, and expensive, to undertake
Willingness to pay allows measurement of potential benefits of health care other than just health gain	It is difficult to assign monetary values to health-care benefits, e.g. oral health improvement

- *Cost-minimization analysis (CMA)* is a fourth type of decision analysis that considers only costs without including consequences of treatment or a health-care programme. Hence, it is not a full economic evaluation. CMA assumes that the two options are equivalent in terms of consequences, but this assumption is very rarely justifiable.

5.3 Practical Approaches to the Economic Evaluation of Teledentistry

As compared to other health-care sectors, economic evaluations are less frequent in oral health care. They are mostly performed on treatment and dental materials and very rarely in preventive dentistry [6]. Basically, the efficiency of teledentistry programmes can be performed either alongside a clinical trial or through modelling methods.

5.3.1 Economic Evaluation Alongside Clinical Trials

Implementing the economic evaluation of teledentistry alongside clinical trials raises two issues: (1) the collection of effectiveness data through a randomized controlled trial and (2) the analysis of these patient-level data.

RCTs have strengths and weaknesses when used for economic evaluation purpose. Collecting effectiveness data alongside an RCT is more relevant in the case of a pragmatic trial, as compared with explanatory ones.

Implementing the economic evaluation of teledentistry alongside an RCT is attractive because it provides patient-level data for both the cost and effectiveness sides and because the marginal cost of collecting cost data is usually modest.

But the following issues are raised:

- Choice of the comparison therapy (i.e. no treatment or current face-to-face practice).
- Outcomes measurement: RCTs usually rely on measurements that are more detailed, invasive and costly than in usual care. Differences in costs and diagnostic accuracy have to be accounted for.
- Intermediate vs. final outcomes: intermediate outcomes (e.g. oral health score or timely appointment rate) are not sufficient in cost-effectiveness evaluations, except if the link with final outcomes (e.g. improved quality of life or survival) has been clearly demonstrated.
- Length of follow-up: the preferred lifelong time horizon might be longer than the follow-up in an RCT.
- Protocol-driven costs and outcomes: one should be able to identify the costs associated with the trial per se, such as the costs due to patient inclusion, informed consent collection, randomization and data collection. Moreover, close and frequent follow-up may result in different health outcomes.
- In real-life use, both physicians and patients do not always strictly conform to the rules mandated by the protocol.

One possibility is to design real-life RCTs, called pragmatic trials. Indeed, inclusion criteria are broader, teledentistry is compared to the current face-to-face care, settings and dentists are representative, follow-up is done under routine conditions and a wide range of endpoints are measured. However, some of the previous problems are retained.

Regardless of the trial type, collecting resource use data is challenging. In teledentistry, relevant costs typically include the teledental device and network infrastructure, staff costs (nurse, dental assistant and dentist), travel costs and training costs [7, 8]. Resource consumption can usually be collected using an adapted case report form (CRF), with the amount of detail depending on the treatment being compared. Data collection can be performed either at the patient level (e.g. staff time), at the facility level (e.g. network infrastructure) or at the programme level (e.g. shared teledentistry devices). However, collecting costs of treatment consequences (e.g. complications or readmissions) is more problematic and may imply the implementation of dedicated solutions, including patient recall (by mail survey or telephone interviews) and access to computerized medical databases.

5.3.1.1 Quantifying Uncertainty in Stochastic Cost-Effectiveness Analysis

Three general approaches can be used to quantify uncertainty in stochastic analysis.

Formal *hypothesis testing* can be performed, the null hypothesis being the absence of difference between treatments and the alternative hypothesis being different outcomes. However, rejecting the alternative hypothesis does not necessarily mean that the null one is true (type II error or lack of power). Clinical trials are often not powered to show a statistical difference in every outcome. However, some people argue that the difference between the means is the best estimate of effect difference rather than zero, rejecting the conventional rules of statistical inference.

Estimation allows reporting confidence intervals ('effect size') rather than only p-values. Calculating confidence intervals using standard formulas based on sample estimates of variance leads to confidence regions (confidence boxes or confidence ellipses), defined as two-dimensional confidence intervals. But confidence regions assume no covariance in cost and effect differences (i.e. no correlation between the differences in costs and the differences in effects) and normally distributed data. These issues can be partially or completely overcome by the Fieller's method and non-parametric bootstrapping. Though not widely used, net monetary benefit can be another way forward. Calculating NMB instead of ICER implies rescaling effectiveness into monetary value using methods based on willingness to pay.

Cost-effectiveness acceptability curves are increasingly used. Using a Bayesian statistical interpretation, CEAC show the probability that, if a treatment is funded, this will be the correct decision. CEAC are usually derived from patient-level effectiveness and cost data through non-parametric bootstrapping.

5.3.2 Economic Evaluation of a Teledentistry Programme Through Modelling

In some instances, implementing an RCT is not feasible or is too costly. In such cases, designing and running a model might be the preferred option.

5.3.2.1 Requirements for Economic Evaluation for Decision-Making

There are two related questions which any health-care system needs to address in making decisions about the cost-effectiveness of a teledentistry programme.

- Can the teledentistry programme be considered cost-effective based on existing evidence (adoption decision)?
- Is it a cost-effective use of resources to demand additional evidence through research (research decision)?

Given these two fundamental questions, a series of requirements for economic evaluation emerges, two of which are related to consistency across different technology appraisals and five others to the economic analyses itself.

- Consistent implementation of the measure of health gain in analyses informing decisions about different technologies (e.g. QALY).
- Consistency in perspective across adoption decisions.
- Appropriate specification of the decision problem—all relevant options need to be defined.
- All relevant evidence.
- Appropriate time horizon—the time period over which costs and benefits are likely to differ between the alternative options.
- Relevant to the decision context.
- Appropriate characterization of uncertainty.

The more appropriate framework for economic analysis is evidence synthesis and decision modelling where all available data are brought to bear on fully specified decision problems [9].

5.3.2.2 Role of Decision-Analytic Models

To compare all relevant options, it is likely that effectiveness data will have to be taken from several trials. Meta-analysis will be necessary to synthesize this type for evidence, but the decision model will provide the framework to combine it with other types of evidence and to allow for head-to-head comparison where randomized clinical trials do not exist.

For economic evaluation, it is not just effectiveness evidence that is required. In addition, all evidence relating to resource use, unit costs, health-related quality of life and the variability around these data are required.

Economic evaluation also requires that intermediate clinical endpoints (e.g. oral health score or timely access to dental care) are linked to health-related quality-of-life data (QALYs).

The appropriate time period for the purpose of an economic evaluation should be long enough to capture in full the differences in resource use, costs and benefits between the alternative options being evaluated. It will be necessary to extrapolate beyond the available clinical data. In theory, the preferred time horizon regarding dental care is lifelong.

With regards to the relevance of the decision context, there might be a mismatch between the available effectiveness data and the actual clinical practice. There might also be a need to adjust data from one setting and location to make it relevant to another jurisdiction. A third example concerns the use of decision models to focus on one or more subgroups; as cost-effectiveness is driven by absolute benefit, a subgroup with a higher baseline risk of an undesirable event will be more cost-effective to treat with a proportional risk reduction intervention.

Decision-analytic models allow for a more thorough characterization of uncertainty and variability.

5.3.2.3 Stages in the Development of a Decision-Analytic Model

The first step is to define the decision problem. It is important to define the range and details of the alternative options (e.g. face-to-face dental care, the recipient population (e.g. the general population, remote population or frail population)) and the location and setting of the interventions being evaluated. The scope and boundaries of the model need to be identified.

The next step is to decide on the appropriate type of decision model to use. The main approaches are decision trees and Markov models.

After that, the available evidence needs to be identified and synthesized. Methods for identifying data should be transparent, and the data itself should be appropriate. As the evidence will likely come from different sources and be of different natures, it will need to be synthesized in a proper way. Multi-parameter evidence synthesis techniques are emerging specifically designed to address health economic decision modelling questions.

Evaluation of the model is a further important step in the development of a decision model and should be centred on the assumptions and model structure, the input parameters and any distributions around them and the output and conclusions. Internal validity relates to the logic of the model and whether the model inputs relate to its outputs. External validation of a model concerns the extent to which the model results can be generalized beyond the evidence used for its development. It checks whether the model can accurately predict future events (predictive validity). Between-model validation is the process by which the model is compared to other independently developed models.

Uncertainty exists in all economic evaluations and has to be appropriately accounted for. The focus is on methodological or structural uncertainty, parameter uncertainty and variability. Variability has sometimes be termed first-order uncertainty and can be defined as the random chance that identical patients will experience different outcomes. Parameter uncertainty can be handled with through univariate sensitivity analysis, multivariate sensitivity analysis and/or probabilistic sensitivity analysis through Monte Carlo simulation. Different distribution curves exist for probabilities, costs, utilities and relative risks. Structural uncertainty is more difficult to deal with and would require the model to incorporate 'competing' structural assumptions with weights representing each assumption's plausibility.

5.3.2.4 Markov Models

Markov models model uncertain events as transitions between health states. They are suited when the timing of events is important and when events may happen more than once, thus when costs and effects are spread over a long period of time, such as in the case of chronic diseases.

It comprises a finite set of health states in which an individual can be found. All individuals in the same health state have the same characteristics. Subjects move between states during a series of cycles of short time intervals, as defined by transition probabilities.

A proper decision has to be made over what time horizon the model needs to run. Costs and benefits need to be attributed to each of the states. State rewards are the values of costs and outcomes assigned to a Markov state. Transition rewards are accrued when there is a cost or outcome related to the transition from one state to another.

Markov models allow the discounting of costs and benefits at the point in time they occur.

In most cases, there might be trend of increasing or decreasing probabilities over time. There might be two types of time dependency: one where the transition probability is linked to age and another where the transition probability is linked to the length of stay in the specific health state.

The Markovian assumption is that all patients in a given health state are homogenous regardless of past health states or how long they have been in that particular state (the Markov model has no memory). This can be overcome by using temporary states and tunnel states. Tunnel states are a series of temporary states that must be visited in a fixed sequence, with each one leading to the next, each representing differing transition probabilities, costs and outcomes.

When the analyst requires memory to be an inherent part of their model, it may be more appropriate to use patient-level simulation models (individual patient sampling or microsimulations). However, these require more evidence and bear more computational burden, especially since a second level of simulation is needed for sensitivity analysis.

5.4 Literature Review

A review published in 2009 identified the research gaps, limitations and challenges associated with the economic evaluation of telemedicine in general [7]:

- Limited generalizability: Given the heterogeneity of telemedicine programmes, most of the results cannot be generalized.
- Disparate estimation methods: There is no uniform methodology or guidelines to conduct standardized economic evaluation in telemedicine.
- Few completed BCAs: Most economic evaluations focus on programme costs and have not deeply researched a broad range of economic benefits from a variety of perspectives.
- Lack of RCTs: The use of RCTs in telemedicine is scant.
- Lack of long-term evaluation studies: Long-term studies in telemedicine are rare so that sustainability of these initiatives cannot be studied.
- Absence of quality data and appropriate measures: Shortage of appropriate data undermines the quality and reliability of economic evaluation.
- Small sample sizes: Telemedicine programmes usually involve small samples, thus posing important statistical limitations.

Although the scope of this review was telemedicine in general, the main findings might hold true for teledentistry.

We conducted a systematic literature search in September 2016 on PubMed using the following search strategy:

'Teledentistry and (cost* OR economic* OR economic OR efficiency)'.

Five articles were retrieved; the main findings are summarized hereafter.

A 12-month trial study was conducted in 2002 in Scotland [10]. The primary objective was to conduct a cost-minimization analysis by comparing the costs of teledentistry with two alternatives: outreach visits and hospital visits. Twenty-five patients were included in two general dental practices in remote settings. The results of this trial study showed that the cost of teledentistry was higher than outreach visits and lower than hospital visits. There were cost savings when patient time was included. The authors suggest that the benefits of teledentistry would be greatest in remote settings and would improve with greater familiarity with equipment.

Peebles HG assessed the cost-effectiveness of the Southeast Health District's school-based teledentistry programme in Georgia as compared to traditional dentistry [11]. In total, 164 children were included in the study. The cost of equipment, personnel, facilities, travel and parents' wages were considered. The teledentistry programme was found to be cost-effective, especially when intangible costs were considered.

An economic analysis of the Total Dental Access teledentistry project within the Department of Defense was published in 1999 [12]. It suggested a return on investment for the current teledentistry system within 1 year of deployment and a return on investment within 6 months for future deployments. However detailed results of this study are not available and their transferability cannot be assessed.

A cost-minimization analysis of two teledentistry models in residential aged care facilities situated in rural areas in Victoria, Australia, was performed [13, 14]. Two models were run on 100 patients to compare an asynchronous treatment plan preparation and a real-time remotely located dental care professional, to the traditional face-to-face model. Direct intervention costs and programme costs were measured. The asynchronous assessment and treatment plan (AU$32 per patient) was the least expensive, followed by the face-to-face model (AU$37 per patient) and by the real-time remote examination (AU$41 per patient). However these differences were not statistically significant.

The last paper reports a cost-effectiveness analysis of implementing teledentistry for rural paediatric patients in Victoria, Australia. From a societal perspective, teledentistry was a dominant strategy compared to face-to-face consultation, resulting in a lower cost (AU$294 vs. AU$431) and a higher rate of timely consultations (70 vs. 66%).

Conclusion

Teledentistry might improve the performance of oral health care in terms of efficiency and equity. By comparing teledentistry programmes to traditional dental care models in terms of their costs and consequences, economic evaluations can help policymakers in identifying and supporting high-value models of care.

However the literature review stresses the paucity of the scientific literature reporting economic evaluations of teledentistry programmes worldwide. In addition, researchers are facing recurrent methodological issues, including the choice of the comparator, the definition of consequences, the time horizon, the inclusion of indirect and intangible costs and the transferability of results.

The way forward might include the foundation of an international scientific network focused on the economics of teledentistry. One of its first achievements could be the writing of methodological guidelines dedicated to the economic evaluation of teledentistry.

References

1. Smith, Peter C., ed. Performance measurement for health system improvement: experiences, challenges and prospects. Cambridge University Press, 2009.
2. Daniel SJ, Kumar S. Comparison of dental hygienists and dentists: clinical and teledentistry identification of dental caries in children. Int J Dent Hyg. 2016;15:e143–8. https://doi.org/10.1111/idh.12232.
3. Drummond M, Sculpher M, Torrance G, O'Brien B, Stoddart G. Methods for the economic evaluation of health care programmes. 3rd ed. Oxford: Oxford University Press; 2005.
4. Murray C, Evans DB, Acharya A, Baltussen R. Development of WHO guidelines on generalized cost-effectiveness analysis. Health Econ. 2000;9:235–51.
5. Mariño R, Ghanim A. Teledentistry: a systematic review of the literature. J Telemed Telecare. 2013;19:189–94.
6. Mariño R, Kahn A, Morgan M. Systematic review of publications on economic evaluations of caries prevention programs. Caries Res. 2013;47:265–72. https://doi.org/10.1159/000346917.
7. Dávalos ME, French MT, Burdick AE, Simmons SC. Economic evaluation of telemedicine: review of the literature and research guidelines for benefit–cost analysis. Telemed e-Health. 2009;15(10):933–48.
8. Kidholm K, Ekeland AG, Jensen LK, Rasmussen J, Pedersen CD, Bowes A, Bech M. A model for assessment of telemedicine applications: mast. Int J Technol Assess Health Care. 2012;28(1):44–51.
9. Mark J. Sculpher, Karl Claxton, Mike Drummond, Chris McCabe. Whither trial-based economic evaluation for health care decision making?. Health Economics 2016;15(7):677–87.
10. Scuffham PA, Steed M. An economic evaluation of the highlands and islands teledentistry project. J Telemed Telecare. 2002;8:165–77.
11. Peebles HG. A cost-effectiveness analysis of the Southeast health district's teledentistry program. Atlanta: Emory University; 2011.
12. Rocca MA, Kudryk VL, Pajak JC, Morris T. The evolution of a teledentistry system within the Department of Defense. Proc AMIA Symp. 1999;1999:921–4.
13. Mariño R, Tonmukayakul U, Manton D, Stranieri A, Clarke K. Cost-analysis of teledentistry in residential aged care facilities. J Telemed Telecare. 2015;22:326–32. https://doi.org/10.1177/1357633X15608991.
14. Mariño R, Tonmukayakul U, Marwaha P, Collmann R, Hopcraft M, Manton D, et al. Teleconsultation/telediagnosis using teledentistry technology: a pilot feasibility study. Int J Adv Life Sci. 2014;6:291–9.

Part II

E-health Care in Oral Medicine

A Clinical Evaluation of Teledentistry in Oral Health Promotion

6

Hans Boeckx

Abstract

The elderly population is increasing proportionally, what calls for new techniques to be adopted in order to sustain the simultaneously growing need for dental evaluation and care. In a serie of preliminary results, conducted in a multicentric study in Belgium by (postgraduate) students, we aim to indicate a more precise view on the aspects of teledentistry in a clinical setting. The assessment was executed using the SoproCare intra-oral camera (Acteon), which allows us to switch between 3 different modes during the scanning protocol. These results were then compared with a simultaneously performed standard clinical examination by another operator and with an extensive questionnaire, conducted by the patient.

Keywords

Teledentistry • Clinical application • Multicentric

H. Boeckx
Master of Science in Dentistry, Postgraduate Student, KU Leuven, Leuven, Belgium
e-mail: hans.boeckx@uzleuven.be

N. Giraudeau (ed.), *e-Health Care in Dentistry and Oral Medicine*,
https://doi.org/10.1007/978-3-319-69450-4_6

6.1 Social Relevance (Introduction)

The absolute number and proportion of elderly is increasing. This trend will continue for the next century. Until 2050, we expect a significant growth in the number of elderly with disabilities. Family or social workers cannot always maintain good home care for this group of people. In that case, a nursing home is often inevitable. In a nursing home, physically or mentally unfit, thus frail elderly can receive care that is both personal and nursing. Registered nurses and caregivers provide this care. The Belgian social system accommodates in remunerated healthcare for elderly, in more than 1600 nursing homes across the country. This is applicable for 257,000 older Belgians (2.4% of the total population), when taking their care dependency into account (on March 31, 2007). Fifty-three percent of these (136,830) had home care support, and 47% (120,170) were living in nursing homes [1].

Oral health must be included in the daily care of the aged people because it is an essential and integral part of general health. It has a severe impact in terms of pain and suffering, impairment of function, and effect on quality of life. Mastication, food selection, weight, speech, taste, hydration, appearance, and psychosocial behavior are influenced by oral health. Thereby it can be seen as a concern not only for the older individuals themselves but also for their family, friends, and healthcare workers [2]. That is why we need to invest in disease control and oral health improvement. The World Oral Health Report 2003 already outlined important principles to do so [3].

Technical advances during the past decades have resulted in a reduced proportion of edentulous individuals. The downside of this positive evolution holds an increased risk for tooth-related oral infections (caries, periodontal disease, endodontic complication, etc.). This asks for an excessive preventive and curative oral healthcare program for older generations, which often isn't included in general health promotion. As a result, oral health problems occur, such as tooth decay (especially root surface decay), gingival/periodontal inflammation, denture-related oral mucosal lesions, and hyposalivation, which often remain underdiagnosed in comparison with general health problems [1], even though studies have shown a clear correlation between systemic diseases and oral health-related problems (e.g., diabetes vs. periodontal disease).

Even when still living at home, we observe weakened oral health due to of self-care neglect, less professional care, and reduced oral health care. At the moment of entering a nursing home, there is already an urgent need of oral healthcare. The situation will deteriorate during the residency because of increasing care dependency and subsequent lack of oral healthcare.

Access to oral consultation is very difficult for the elderly in nursing homes in Belgium.

A study of the socialistic mutuality investigated the dental care of 65+ in nursing homes. They analyzed the data of 18.000 members and compared them with a control group of 65+ who still lives at home [4]. The results were as follows. More than three on four inhabitants haven't seen a dentist over a period of 2 years. Twenty-two percent has not had any form of dental care. Another observation is a relation between age and number of dental visits. The older the inhabitants, the less dental care they get (26% at age 65–74 years and 20% at age 85+). Dental care is also related to dependency to others help. The more reliant upon others care, the less dental care. The study also concluded that the people who still live at home get more dental care than the inhabitants of a nursing home.

We can think of some reasons to explain this observation.

1. Older people have less teeth so accordingly less need of dental care.
2. The attention for oral healthcare of the caregivers is limited.
3. Transportation of a less mobile or confused inhabitant to a dentist is not to be underestimated.
4. Dental care can be expensive and is one of the first things on which inhabitants will try to save.
5. A lot of inhabitants are not able anymore to tell their problems and needs, so it is difficult to help them.

Furthermore, as people in Flanders grow older, the population of dentists also does. In 2003, nearly one-fifth (18.4%) of all dentists were younger than 35 years, one-third were between 36 and 45 years, and nearly half of them (48.5%) were older than 45. Another finding is a gradual feminization of the dental profession. In Flanders, 43.4% of all dentists were women in 2003. We see a difference in goals and ways of working between male and female dentists. Female dentists pay in general more attention to preventive dentistry.

As support to achieve this, we can also do consultations at a distance. Thus, we can estimate care needs in persons with compromised mobility. The intraoral camera SoproCare of the company Acteon provides high accuracy with strong image magnification for the visibility of lesions in the order of millimeters. Furthermore, this camera uses autofluorescence that allows to highlight oral plaque, early caries, and gingival inflammations [4].

The objective of this study is to validate the teledentistry system, which consists of the SoproCare camera combined with software that registers, processes, and communicates oral health-related information. This validation implies comparison of information obtained with the teledentistry system with information obtained from the gold standard, namely, a clinical oral assessment.

6.2 Materials and Methods

6.2.1 Objectives

The main objectives in assessing the validity of the teledentistry system as a diagnostic tool were *oral hygiene, presence of calculus, dental caries, periodontal health,* and *oral mucosa health*. The results were simultaneously compared to conventional clinical oral examinations. In addition, an extensive questionnaire was linked to each evaluation, so we could search for other correlations. Those secondary objectives consisted of: correspondence between caries seen during visual examination and caries seen during SoproCare examination (A), difference between the gradation of caries at visual examination and the gradation of caries at SoproCare examination (B), gingivitis index measured at visual examination compared to the index at SoproCare examination (C), time needed to do SoproCare examination (filming + interpretation) compared to time needed for visual examination (D), plaque index measured during visual examination compared to the index during SoproCare examination (E), relationship between calculus and gingivitis index (F), relationship between pain and caries (G), correspondence between soft tissue lesions seen during visual examination and soft tissue lesions during SoproCare examination (H), soft tissue lesions seen during visual examination related to pain (I), mental and physical cooperation during visual examination compared to SoproCare examination (J), patients feedback of visual examination compared to feedback of SoproCare examination (K), examiners feedback of visual examination compared to SoproCare examination (L), dry mouth and bad breath (M), subjective rating of oral health (N), presence of pain (O), satisfaction concerning dentures (P), chewing comfort (Q), and need of care (R).

6.2.2 Research Protocol

Benefits of the teledentistry approach is the expected improvement of access to care of care-dependent individuals, often with limited mobility, because it allows the dentist to indicate whether this person should visit a dentist or the dentist should go to the patient in the nursing home. Moreover, it avoids devious transportation measurements (accompanying staff required, expensive, patient discomfort, etc.) and could allow peer discussion among fellow dental caretakers to better facilitate treatment planning. Inevitable risks are a chance of underdiagnosis of oral pathology and potential worsening of non-detected pathology caused by delay of dental visitation.

6.2.3 Research Design

This single-center, blinded study was conducted as a cross-sectional census that evaluates a cohort of 100 elderlies (above the age of 65) to validate a diagnostic device. Before starting the feasibility study, researchers will have a basic training to learn the use of the SoproCare camera. KU Leuven staff provided training and technical support in digital photography. The first examination (following gold-standard procedures) was executed by a senior dental student, while a second examination (with the SoproCare camera) was performed separately by another senior dental student. [5]

6.2.3.1 Gold Standard

Evaluation of Patients Concerns

The patient is provided with a questionnaire depending on the overall oral condition, consisting of questions either based on the presence of only natural teeth, only dentures, or a combination.

These questions were:

- Are you experiencing any pain or discomfort? (No/Yes, specify)
- Are there any overall complaints? (No/Yes, specify)
- Do you have certain wishes? (No/Yes, specify)
- Do you suffer from a dry mouth? (No/Yes, specify)
- How do you describe your chewing comfort? (Adequate/Not adequate)
- Are you experiencing any tooth mobility (No/Yes)?
- How do you judge the condition of your teeth? (Bad/Moderate/Good/Excellent)
- How do you clean your denture(s)?
- Do you use any chemical agent to clean your denture(s)? (No/Yes, specify)
- How frequently do you clean your denture(s)? (Numeric answer)
- How old are your denture(s)? (Numeric answer)
- Are you satisfied with your denture(s)? (Yes/No, specify)

Caries Detection

Due to the logistic limitation on site (only proper lighting, a dental probe and a mirror), we maintained an adjusted version of the ICDAS [5, 6] reference for scaling carious lesions. The ICDAS *(International Caries Detection and Assessment System)* consists of two digits, each covering a specific description of the carious lesion. The first digit indicates the "surface condition," while the second refers to the "carious type" [7].

First digit	Second digit
0: Not restored or sealed	Code 0: sound
1: Partially sealed	Code 1: visual change in enamel, seen dry
2: Fully sealed	Code 2: distinct visual change in enamel, seen wet or dry. Carious opacity (white spot lesion) or discoloration (brown spot lesion) that is wider than the natural fissure or fossa and is inconsistent with sound enamel
3: Tooth colored restoration	Code 3: localized enamel breakdown, no dentin visible
4: Amalgam restoration	Code 4: underlying dark shadow of discolored dentin visible through intact enamel. More noticeable when the surface is wet
5: Stainless steel crown	Code 5: distinct cavity with visible dentin. When wet, darkening of the dentin may be visible through the enamel. When dry, tooth structure loss and demineralization can be seen at the pit of fissure. On smooth surfaces, it involves less than half of the tooth structure
6: Porcelain/gold/PFM crown	Code 6: extensive distinct cavity with visible dentin involving at least half of the tooth surface or the pulp (can be deep and wide)
7: Lost or broken restoration	Code 7: only a root is visible, affected by caries
8: Temporary restoration	

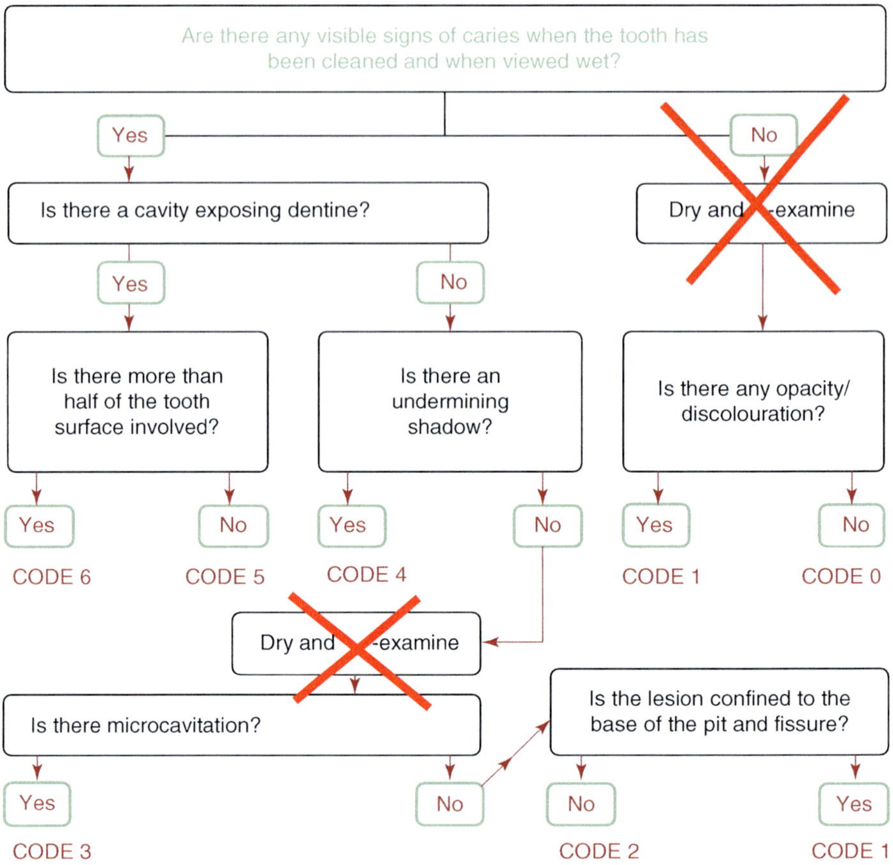

Because of the lack of extensive equipment, we adjusted the regular ICDAS examination protocol to our means, which we indicated in *italic*.

(a) Ask patient to remove any removable appliances
We did the same. In addition, we wrote down the overall condition of the appliance.
(b) Clean the appliance
We skipped this part
(c) Place cotton wool in buccal vestibules
We skipped this part, the tooth surfaces do not need to be dry in our protocol
(d) Remove excess/frothy saliva
We skipped this part, we only have access to light/probe/mirror
(e) Visual examination of the wet surface
We did the same, already providing a score in this step
(f) Dry the surface for 5 s

We skipped this part, surface didn't need to be dry in our protocol

(g) Visual inspection of the dry surface, no probing
Not applicable because no dry surfaces are needed

(h) Do not use a probe, only ball-ended can be gently used
We decided to use a probe in our examination

Plaque Index

To determine the plaque index, we use the modified Navy plaque index [8] to describe the presence or absence of plaque. We could use the Ramfjord elements, but the staff of the nursing homes might not understand the meaning of that. It is also possible that they do not know what to do when some of the Ramfjord elements are missing. For that reason, we will use all the present teeth.

How do we use this index?

We will separate the teeth in eight planes (four vestibular and four lingual/palatal as on the picture):

- No plaque = 0
- Plaque not in contact with the gingiva = 1
- Plaque strictly vestibular or palatal/lingual in contact with the gingiva = 2
- Plaque mesial or distal of the teeth in contact with the gingiva = 3
- We will sum all the values and divide them by the number of received values. The obtained value is plaque index. When under 0.6 (or 0.6), the oral hygiene is good; when over 0.6, the oral hygiene is bad. In this case, we should encourage and motivate the patient and explain how to brush better.

In the clinic, we use erythrosine red to reveal where the plaque is located. We will coat the teeth and let the patient rinse until the water spit out is colorless. When some of the surfaces stay colored, it indicates plaque. We show this to the patient in a mirror. This way the patient knows where to clean better. In the nursing homes, we will not use erythrosine red because we do not have the possibilities to polish the teeth whereby it may be impossible to remove all the red discoloration. Instead we will look at the teeth and feel with our probe to reveal the present plaque.

Denture Plaque

Loose debris is rinsed off the denture. Plaque will not be removed by rinsing the denture. Accumulations on the dentures are divided into eight groups, four on the vestibular surface and four on the palatal surface. The scoring is done and the results are scored as following:

0. No plaque
1. Light plaque, 1–25% of area covered
2. Moderate plaque, 26–50% of area covered
3. Heavy plaque, 51–75% of area covered
4. Very heavy plaque, 76–100% of area covered

- We have not looked at the plaque on the dentures because it was too devious to do that. Most of the dentures were very unclean caused by eating remnants. We also checked the dentures for fractures.

Calculus

We used a simple Yes/No indication: "Yes" if scaling was needed; "No" if no scaling was needed.

Posterior Occluding Couples of Teeth

Gives information about chewing comfort. We just counted the couples while the patient was occluding. Figures went from a minimum of 0 to a maximum of 6.

Gingivitis Index

Since we cannot probe while using the SoproCare camera, we score according to what we can see in the mouth.

1. Healthy gingiva
2. Moderate infected gingiva
3. Severely infected gingiva

Soft Tissue Lesions

Yes, if a soft tissue lesion is present. If "yes" we will name the lesion.
No if there is no soft tissue lesion.

Experience + Feedback Patient

0 = the patient is very annoyed. He is not willing to do this ever again
1 = the patient finds the examination not pleasant but understands the importance and is willing to do this later again.
2 = the patient had a rather pleasant experience and is grateful.

Experience + Feedback Researcher

0 = the examination went very difficult; we had to make some compromises and did not do everything like the protocol description.
1 = the examination went difficult, but it was possible to get the results accordingly to the protocol description.
2 = the examination went very good. We could work efficiently and get the results accordingly to the protocol description.

Compliance Patient

Mental

0 = patient is not willing to cooperate (e.g., dementia in advanced stage).
1 = it took some effort to convince the patient to cooperate (e.g., a distrusting patient), but it was possible to do our research.
2 = There were no mental limitations.

We will try to select only patients with mental compliance of score 1 or 2.

Physical
0 = patient is not able to cooperate due to physical limitations (e.g., opening of the mouth).
1 = it took some effort, but it was possible to do our research (e.g., difficulties concerning the opening of the mouth and a need for closing the mouth from time to time).
2 = there were no physical limitations.
We will try to select only patients with physical compliance of score 1 or 2.

Time Needed to Do the Oral Examination
We will measure the time needed to do all steps, discussed in Sect. 6.4.1.1 from point "b" till "h."

(We will not measure time for questionnaire, feedback, and compliance rating.)

This way, we can evaluate our progress in efficiency. We can also compare the time needed to do the gold-standard exam with the time needed to do the scanning with the SoproCare camera.

6.2.3.2 Teledentistry System

Diagnostics will be made using the SoproCare camera of the Acteon company. The images will be read by a remote operator who is different from the hygienist performing the consultation, and its findings will be compared to those of the latter. The SoproCare intraoral camera is used to image the oral hard and soft tissues. Three different working modes are available: daylight mode (only magnification), caries mode (visualization of caries), and perio-mode (visualization of infectious problems of the soft tissues and the presence of plaque or calculus). We will use the software of Acteon while working with the SoproCare.

First, we will explain our protocol of video-making:

1. If the patient has any removable appliances, we ask him to remove them.
2. If the patient has natural teeth:
   Scan the teeth from quadrant 1 till quadrant 4.
   Each quadrant we will begin to scan in cario-mode from posterior to anterior, and then we will return in perio-mode from anterior to posterior. First vestibular and then occlusal and palatal. We will have a total of 24 videos to record all the teeth surfaces if the patient has teeth in each quadrant
3. If the patient is edentulous:
   In case of presence of denture(s), we make a video of the denture(s). We decided not to give a score with the denture plaque index (see paragraph d about denture plaque).
4. Scan the soft tissue in daylight mode.
   We will make a video of the palate and the mouth floor and the alveolar ridge.

If the researcher sees something suspicious, it is possible to make an extra picture.

A SoproCare evaluation includes roughly the same parameters when using the gold standard, yet with small but significant adaptations:

Evaluation of Patient Concerns

The questionnaire is the same as with the conventional examination. The patient only must fill in this form once. The questions can be found in section "Evaluation of Patients Concerns".

Caries Detection

We will scan all teeth with the SoproCare in caries mode, in accordance to our video-making protocol. Afterward the videos will be evaluated by the third dental student who participates the study. Caries are clearly revealed by the bright red color in the cario-mode. Other surrounding tissue is displayed in black and white, thus drawing the focus only to the carious lesion. General assessment is made using the same ICDAS references as in section "Caries Detection".

Plaque Index

To determine the plaque index, we will turn on the perio-mode in accordance to our video-making protocol. Afterward the videos will be evaluated by the third dental student who participates the study. The wavelength emitted by the LED lights of SoproCare highlights the different tissues represented by a chromatic mapping. Gingival inflammation can range from hues of pink all the way to deep magenta. New plaque is highlighted by its white and grainy characteristics, and old plaque is revealed as shades of yellow and orange [9]. The wavelength emitted by the LED lights of SoproCare highlights the different tissues represented by a chromatic mapping. Gingival inflammation can range from hues of pink all the way to deep magenta. We used the same scaling index as in section "Plaque Index".

Denture Plaque

We only scan the dentures in daylight mode. Since it was too devious to do a plaque index on dentures during the gold standard, it is not useful to do one with the SoproCare as we cannot compare both. Furthermore, the same reference scale is used as in section "Denture Plaque".

Calculus

To determine the presence or absence of calculus, we will use perio-mode, although it is also possible to see calculus in daylight mode.

Posterior Occluding Couples of Teeth

While the patient is occluding, it is possible to take a picture or video to assess the amount of occluding pairs.

Gingivitis Index

We will scan the mouth in perio-mode. The third dental student will evaluate the videos and give a score to what he sees. Since we cannot probe, we make a gradation according to what we can see.

1. Healthy gingiva
2. Moderately infected gingiva
3. Severely infected gingiva

The disadvantage of the SoproCare is that we cannot probe, only scan. Consequently, it is not possible to determine the DPSI either.

Soft Tissue Lesions

A video of the soft tissues is made in daylight mode (palate, mouth floor, and alveolar ridge). It is possible to make an extra picture if we see something abnormal. When necessary the dentist can ask for a new picture within a few days to follow the evolution of the lesion.

Daylight mode provides magnification of up to 115 times, revealing details otherwise not visible to the naked eye. This allows close monitoring of soft tissues lesions.

1. Experience + Feedback Patient (See section "Experience + Feedback Patient")
2. Experience + Feedback Researcher (See section "Experience + Feedback Researcher")
3. Compliance Patient (See section "Compliance Patient")

Time Needed to Collect Information with SoproCare

We will measure the time needed to do all the steps, discussed in Sect. 6.4.1.1, from point b till h. We will not measure time for questionnaire, feedback, and compliance rating. This way, we can evaluate our progress in efficiency. We can also compare the time for scanning with SoproCare with the time to do the gold standard. The time to interpret the videos is measured separately.

Time Needed to Interpret Information from SoproCare Evaluation

We will measure the time needed to see and interpret all videos. This way, we can evaluate our progress in efficiency. We can also compare the results in the end with the time needed to do the standard examination.

6.2.3.3 Visit and Examination Provided

Participation of nursing homes is proposed by email. If the nursing home is willing to participate, an appointment is made and further information is given. The nursing home will also sign a letter of support where they confirm their interest in the project. Individual participants need to sign an informed consent after being fully informed (see appendix). One copy will go to the examiners, and one copy and the information brochure are given for their own administration. An examiner will first record photos and videos with the SoproCare camera, and the classic consultation is realized by a different examiner. The participation in this research requires only a single visit. The photos and videos will be diagnosed by a third examiner. The results of both the examinations will be compared to see the extent to which they correspond.

6.2.3.4 Number of Patients + Method of Recruitment

There was a total of 96 patients (spread over the different participating nursing homes). The subjects will be recruited during visits to the institutions for older persons. The participation is completely voluntary. If later the subjects decide to withdraw from the study, it is possible at any time, without having to give a reason and without affecting the future medical care.

6.2.3.5 Criteria for Inclusion

Subjects are eligible to be included in the study if they reside in an institution for older persons

- The subject is more than 65 years old, regardless of gender, ethnic origin, or race.
- The subject must be mentally able to provide informed consent.
- The subject must be physically able to cooperate.

	Center 1		Center 2		Center 3		Center 4		Total	
	N	*%*	*N*	*%*	*N*	*%*	*N*	*%*	*N*	*%*
Gender										
Male	20	44.4	10	45.5	2	25	4	19	36	37.5
Female	25	55.6	12	54.5	6	75	17	81	60	62.5
Total	45	100	22	100	8	100	21	100	96	100
Natural teeth										
Yes	17	37.8	14	63.6	8	100	20	95.2	59	61.5
No	28	62.2	8	36.4	0	0	1	4.8	37	38.5
Total	45	100	22	100	8	100	21	100	96	100

6.2.3.6 Criteria for Exclusion

Subjects will be excluded from the study if they do not meet the abovementioned criteria and/or if they meet the following exclusion criteria:

- The subject for which it is impossible to understand and sign the informed consent.
- The presence of bad physical health interfering with cooperation.

6.2.3.7 Criteria for Ending the Participation in the Study

- Withdrawal of consent
- Decreased mental and physical ability interfering with cooperation

6.3 Results

Because of final statistics still being performed, we decided to preliminary analyze the results by assuming a normal distribution of data.

6.3.1 Correspondence Between Caries Seen During SoproCare and Visual Examination

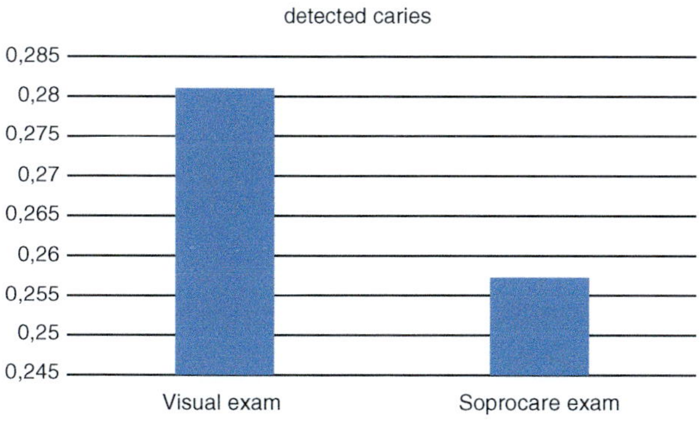

- Mean caries detected at visual exam: 0.28 ± 0.45
- Mean caries detected at SoproCare exam: 0.26 ± 0.44
- T-test: P-value = 0.095, P-value > 0.05 ($\alpha = 5\%$)
  - More caries is detected with visual examination compared to SoproCare system, although the results are not statistically significant.
  - *We noticed that SoproCare examination didn't highlight all the caries. Calculus on the other hand was often colored red in cario-mode due to the presence of porphyrins. Logically the scoring depends also on the quality of the video.*

6.3.2 Difference Between the Gradation of Caries with SoproCare and Visual Examination

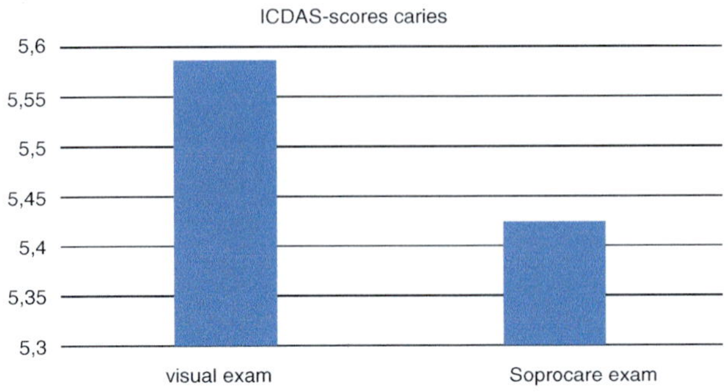

- Mean ICDAS scores made during visual exam: 5.59 ± 1.20
- Mean ICDAS scores made during SoproCare: 5.43 ± 1.25
- T-test: P-value = 0.95, P-value > 0.05 ($\alpha = 5\%$)
  - During SoproCare exam the ICDAS score is lower compared to visual examination, although results are not statistically significant.
  - *We noticed that evaluating the videos we gave a lower ICDAS score compared to looking in the mouth, the caries was often not highlighted in red, or there was only red at one spot in an otherwise clinically extensive lesion. Logically the scoring depends also on the quality of the video.*

6.3.3 Gingivitis Index Measured With SoproCare Versus Visual Examination

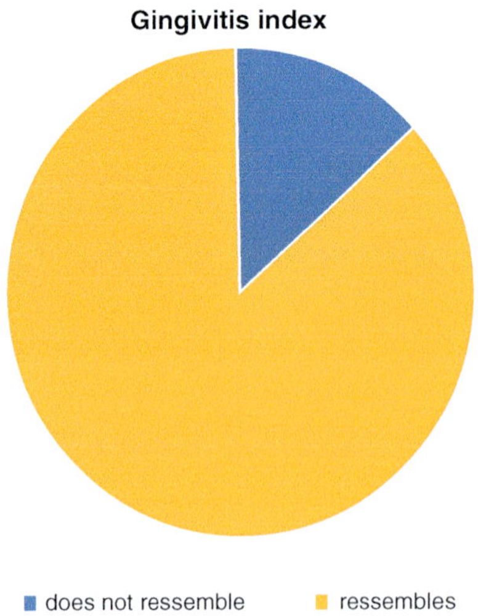

In 86.3% of cases, gingivitis indices are equal. In 13.7% of cases, gingivitis indices differ.

– *We did not notice a big difference between evaluating gingivitis index with or without the camera.*

6.3.4 Time Needed to do SoproCare Examination Compared to Visual Examination

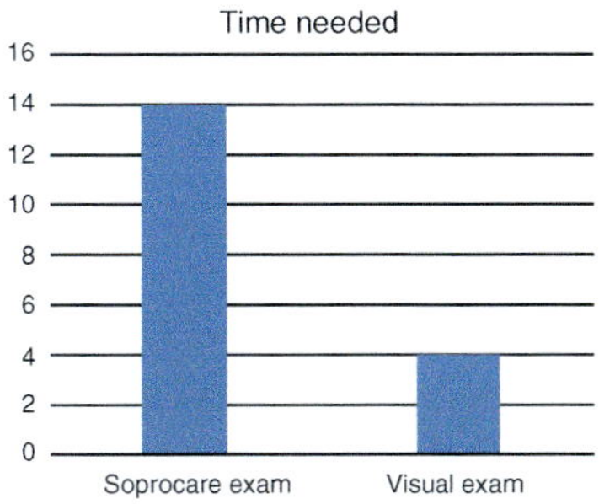

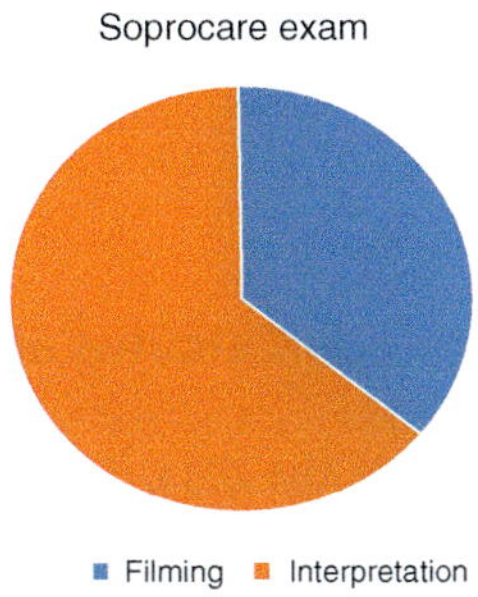

- Mean time needed to perform visual exam: 4 ± 2.82 min
- Mean time needed to perform SoproCare exam (filming + interpreting): 14 ± 11.31 min
  - Whereof filming: 5 ± 2.83 min
  - Whereof interpreting: 9 ± 8.49 min
- T-test: P-value = 1.20×10^{-16}, P-value < 0.05 ($\alpha = 5\%$)
  - SoproCare exam needs a lot more time than visual exam. The time for interpreting is also included. More time is needed for interpretation compared to the filming itself. The results are statistically significant.
  - We noticed that filming with SoproCare was very time-consuming. This was especially applicable when a lot of teeth were present. When edentulous it did not take much time.

6.3.5 Plaque Index Measuring in SoproCare Compared to Visual Examination

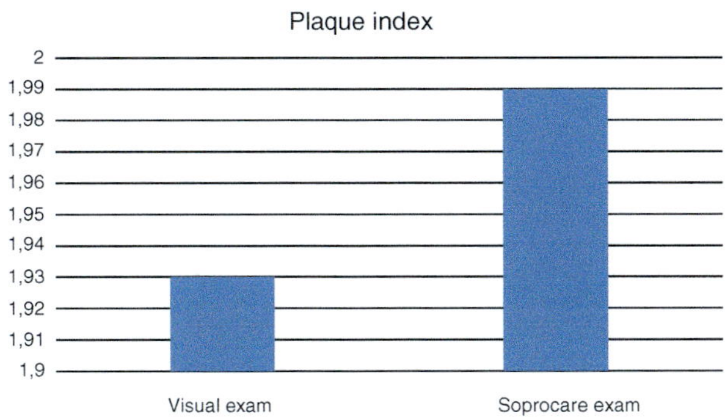

- Mean plaque index at visual exam: 1.93 ± 0.54.
- Mean plaque index at SoproCare exam: 1.99 ± 0.26.
- H_0 = There is a difference between plaque indices score during standard exam compared to SoproCare exam.
- T-test: P-value = 0.43, P-value > 0.05 ($\alpha = 5\%$) ≥ we do not have enough evidence to conclude that H_0 is most probably wrong.
  - Statistically, we cannot say that there is a significant difference between plaque indices during standard exam compared to SoproCare exam.
  - Evaluating the plaque index without erythrosine red was difficult. Especially at visual exam, the scoring was very subjective. The SoproCare camera highlights the plaque in perio-mode and is therefore more accurate.

6.3.6 Relationship Between Calculus and Gingivitis Index

We used a Fisher test to analyze the data. First, we inserted the gingivitis scores made at visual exam and second, the gingivitis scores made at SoproCare exam.

6.3.6.1 Visual Exam (VE)

VE	GI = 1	GI = 2	GI = 3	GI = 4
Presence of calculus	5	33	10	48
Absence of calculus	4	4	0	8
Total	9	37	10	56

H_0 = Patients with and without calculus do have the same distribution of gingivitis index scored at visual exam. Fisher test: 0.022, P-value > 0.05 ($\alpha = 5\%$) ≥ we can reject H_0.

- The patients with and without calculus have different distributions of gingivitis index. This is statistically significant.

6.3.6.2 SoproCare Exam

SE	GI = 1	GI = 2	GI = 3	GI = 4
Presence of calculus	5	32	11	48
Absence of calculus	3	4	0	7
Total	8	36	11	55

H_0 = Patients with and without calculus do have the same distribution of gingivitis index scored at SoproCare exam. Fisher test: 0.071, P-value > 0.05 ≥ we do not have enough evidence to conclude that H_0 is most probably wrong

- We cannot conclude a difference in distribution between patients with and without calculus.

We noticed mostly a correlation between calculus and gingivitis index. This makes sense because the calculus irritates the gums and will cause inflammation.

6.3.7 Relationship Between Pain and Caries

6.3.7.1 With Caries Present at Visual Exam (VE)

VE	ICDAS 4	ICDAS 5	ICDAS 6	ICDAS 7	No caries	Total
Pain present	4	6	4	3	2	19
Pain absent	23	20	17	20	8	88
Total	27	26	21	23	10	107

H_0 = No relationship between pain and caries is present at visual exam.
Fisher test: P-value = 0.886, P-value > 0.05 ($\alpha = 5\%$)

- We do not have enough evidence to conclude that H_0 is most probably wrong. Statistically, we cannot say with 95% certainty that there is a relationship between pain and caries present at visual exam.
- We noticed that patients often did not have pain but had a lot of caries in the mouth. In general the elderly have less sensitive teeth. They often do not go to a dentist when having pain. In time the pain can reduce.

6.3.7.2 With Caries Present at SoproCare Exam

SE	ICDAS 4	ICDAS 5	ICDAS 6	ICDAS 7	No caries	Total
Pain present	6	7	3	3	2	21
Pain absent	23	24	7	18	7	79
Total	29	31	10	21	9	107

H_0 = No relationship between pain and caries is present at SoproCare exam.
Fisher test: P-value = 0.8789, P-value > 0.05 ($\alpha = 5\%$). We do not have enough evidence to conclude that H_0 is most probably wrong.

- Statistically, we cannot say with 95% certainty that there is a relationship between pain and caries present at SoproCare exam.
- We noticed that patients often did not have pain but had a lot of caries in the mouth. In general elderly have less sensitive teeth. They often do not go to a dentist when having pain. In time the pain will often reduce.

6.3.8 Correspondence Between Soft Tissue Lesions During SoproCare Versus Visual Exvam

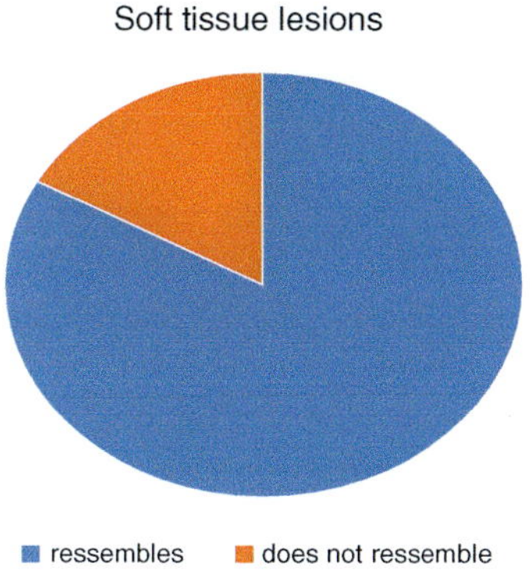

- The kind of lesions are not discussed, only the presence of some lesion in the mouth.
- In 83.2% soft tissue lesions were found in both examinations. In 16.8% there was no correspondence between soft tissue lesions found at different examinations.
- We noticed that evaluating the presence of soft tissue lesions depends on the quality of the videos. If the videos were made very quickly, there is a possibility to miss the lesions. *On the other hand, we could play the video a couple times and in slow motion.*

6.3.9 Soft tissue Lesions Seen During Visual Exam Related to Pain

	Soft tissue lesions VE	No soft tissue lesions VE	Soft tissue lesions SE	No soft tissue lesions SE	Total
Pain present	6	10	4	12	32
Pain absent	36	43	30	49	158
Total	42	53	34	61	190

H_0 = No relationship between soft tissue lesions and pain are present at visual and SoproCare exam. Fisher test: P-value = 0.74, P-value > 0.05 ($\alpha = 5\%$). We do not have enough evidence to conclude that H_0 is most probably wrong.

- Statistically, we cannot say with 95% certainty that there is a relationship between soft tissue lesions and pain during visual exam and SoproCare exam.
- We noticed that if patients say they have pain of their dentures, we could almost always find a soft tissue lesion in the mouth.

6.3.10 Mental and Physical Cooperation During SoproCare Versus Visual Exam

	Mental cooperation VE	Mental cooperation SE	Physical cooperation VE	Physical cooperation SE	Total
0	1	1	0	0	2
1	2	3	5	5	15
2	92	91	90	90	363
Total	95	95	95	95	380

H_0 = There is no difference in mental and physical cooperation during visual exam compared to SoproCare exam. Chi-squared test, P-value = 0.6737164, while Fisher test, P-value = grand total > 100 (380) for 6 df. Fisher test was difficult to evaluate because the values were too high.

- There is no significant difference in cooperation during visual and SoproCare exam.
- We noticed that patients cooperated the same at the two examinations.

6.3.11 Patient Feedback of Visual Examination Compared to SoproCare Protocol

H_0 = Patient feedback is not different for visual exam compared to SoproCare exam. In 90 cases, we see no difference in the feedback when evaluating visual exam or SoproCare exam.

- We cannot apply a statistical test, because the number of disagreements is too small (0). In a case like this, the distribution often cannot be estimated.
- We noticed that the patients gave mostly a good feedback undergoing the SoproCare exam. The feedback of SoproCare exam was mostly equal to the feedback of the visual exam.

6.3.12 Examiners Feedback of Visual Examination Compared to SoproCare Protocol

In 98 cases, examiners give the same score of feedback evaluating visual exam or SoproCare exam

- We cannot apply a statistical test, because the number of disagreements is too small [2]. In a case like this, the distribution often cannot be estimated.
- In general, operating the camera was not that difficult; however, some patients did not cooperate very well.

6.3.13 Dry Mouth and Bad Breath

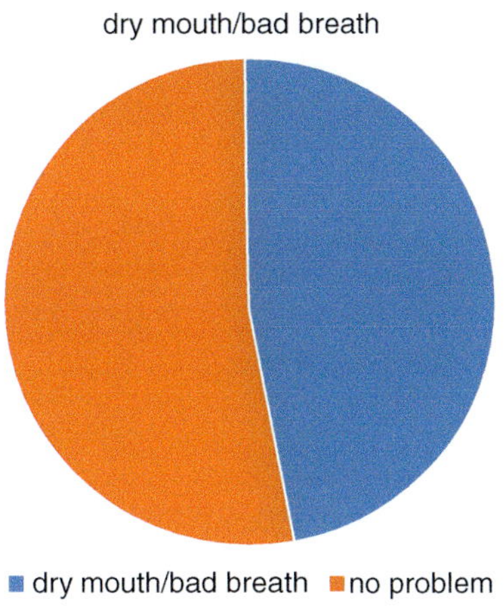

- Inhabitants claiming to have a dry mouth or bad breath: 46.9%
- Inhabitants claiming to have no problems regarding dry mouth/bad breath: 53.1%

- The questionnaire reveals that almost half of the inhabitants complains about having a dry mouth or bad breath. Different factors can contribute to this, but medication plays an important role in the problem.
- We cannot state this statistically

6.3.14 Subjective Rating of Oral Health

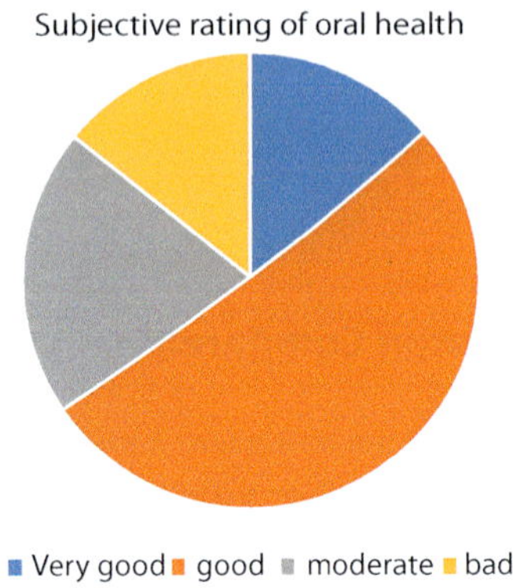

We asked the inhabitants with teeth for a subjective rating of their oral health.

- Very good: 13.8%
- Good: 51.7%
- Moderate: 20.7%
- Bad: 13.8%
  - We noticed that the inhabitants often rated their oral health better than the reality suggested.
  - We cannot state this statistically.

6.3.15 Presence of Pain

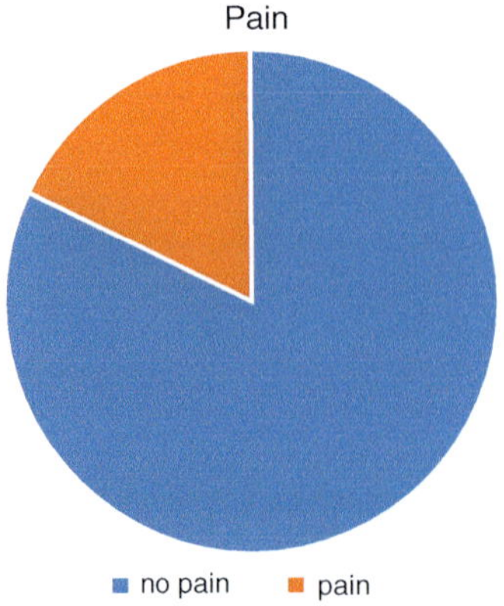

We asked the inhabitants with teeth for a subjective rating of their oral health.

- Very good: 13.8%
- Good: 51.7%
- Moderate: 20.7%
- Bad: 13.8%
  - We noticed that the inhabitants often rated their oral health better than the reality suggested.
  - We cannot state this statistically.

6.3.16 Satisfaction About Denture(s)

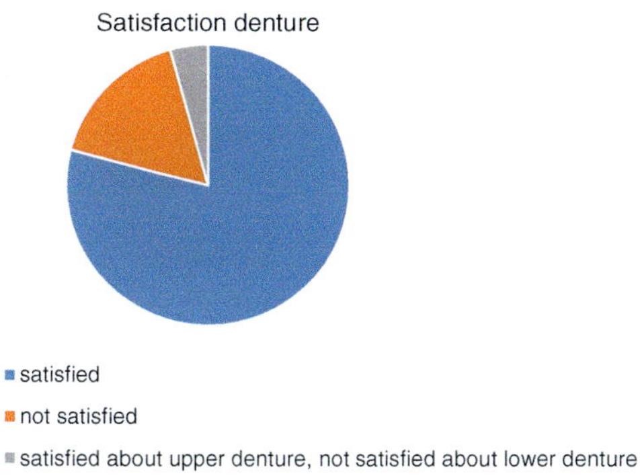

We asked the inhabitants with denture(s) if they are satisfied about them.

- 78% is happy about their denture(s).
- 17% is not happy about their denture(s).
- 4% is happy about the maxillary denture but not about the mandibular denture.
  - We noticed that the inhabitants often do not wish to have new dentures, even when they complain about it.
  - We cannot state this statistically.

6.3.17 Chewing Comfort

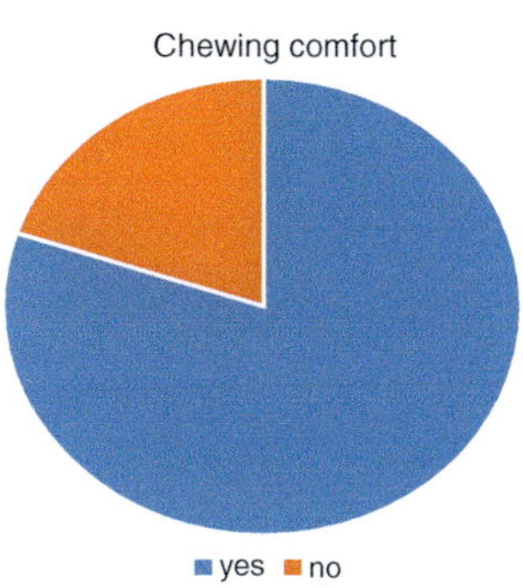

We asked the inhabitants about their chewing comfort.

- 80.2% is satisfied about their chewing comfort. This means that they do not have any difficulties when eating.
- 19.8% has difficulties when eating.
  - We noticed that most inhabitants are satisfied about their chewing comfort.
  - We cannot state this statistically.

6.3.18 Need of Care

We made a treatment plan based on what we saw in the visual exam.

- 21% did not need any treatment or care.
- 79% needed some form of treatment or care. Of this group:
- 8% needed only cleaning.
- 1.3% needed only conservative care.
- 5.3% needed only extractions.
- 2.7% had only a problem regarding the soft tissue.
- 0.4% needed only new dentures.
- 37.3% needed cleaning + conservative care.
- 10.7% needed cleaning + conservative care + extraction.
- 2.7% needed cleaning + conservative care + soft tissue lesions.
- 1.3% needed cleaning + soft tissues lesions + new denture(s).
- 2.7% needed cleaning + conservative care + extractions + new denture(s).
- 2.7% needed extraction + new denture(s).
- 6.7% needed soft tissue lesions + adaptation of denture(s).
- 13.3% needed only adaptation of denture(s).
- 1.3% needed cleaning + adaptation of denture(s).
  - The necessity of care is very high in this group of people.
  - We cannot state this statistically.

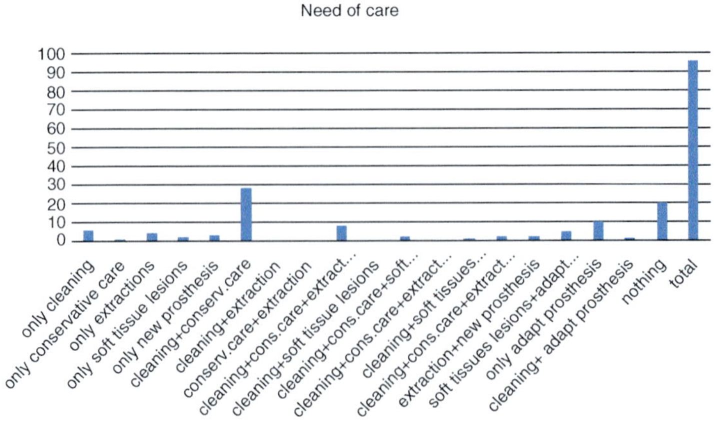

6.4 Discussion

6.4.1 Methods and Materials

First, we will discuss the weaknesses and aberrations of our ideal protocol. We started focusing on the methods and materials we used. The intention was to perform the study according to the research protocol. Evaluating our questionnaire, we noticed that the inhabitants sometimes gave contradictory answers. For instance, some people without teeth but with dentures say to have pain but claim at the same time to be happy about their dentures. Another example is when they say to have pain and give a lot of complaints but also give a very good subjective score to their own teeth.

The question "Do you have pain?" was too vague. It would have been better to make a distinction between different kinds of pain (teeth, soft tissue, or denture). To process this question statistically, it is also better to have a score on a pain scale. For example, let the patient draw a point on a visual line on a paper. Left means no pain, and right means maximum of pain. This is more accurate than asking a number or yes/no. We can say the same about scoring the mental and physical cooperation and feedback. A more accurate way of scoring is needed to make good conclusions.

We asked a lot of questions in the questionnaire but lack some question to make other interesting conclusions. For example, we asked about dry mouth or bad breath but did not ask about medication or smoking. The only thing we can state is that almost half the inhabitants complain about having a dry mouth/bad breath.

Like most researches, the sample of patients in our research was not randomly selected. We contacted some nursing homes and selected patients with good mental and physic capacities. The selected patients needed to sign an informed consent. We tried to convince the inhabitants to cooperate but did not push anyone. The sample is not random and thereby probably not representative. We also noticed a big difference in results when conducting the research in one nursing home compared to another. For example, nursing homes collaborating with social services counted more edentulous people with dentures. On the other hand, inhabitants of service flats had a lot of teeth.

Our goal to have a sample of 100 elderlies was almost reached. We did our research on 96 patients. But even if we could have reached our goal of 100 patients, this sample is still too restricted. It would be more accurate and representative to have a bigger sample. In one center, we noticed that a great number of inhabitants in the nursing home were edentulous. To compensate this, in the other nursing homes, we selected only inhabitants with teeth to have a more representative balance.

We have done our visual examination in the room of the inhabitants so the circumstances to detect problems were far from ideal. The only light source we had was a flashlight, and we had to stand or sit in a difficult position. Moreover, most of the inhabitants had so much plaque or eating remnants, so it was not possible to detect all the caries. Experience tells us that if you want to do an accurate examination, the first thing to do is a cleaning.

We wanted to color the plaque of the patients with erythrosine, but practically this was infeasible. We decided to estimate the presence of plaque by sight. Considering plaque has a white color, we probably have missed some, resulting in a less accurate scoring.

The disadvantage of doing the research with three students is the inevitable difference in scoring and evaluating. We tried to harmonize our techniques and scoring as much as possible but did not have a calibration test.

6.4.1.1 This Part Will Handle Difficulties Using SoproCare

A silicon cap is applicable on the camera to filter and avoid detrimental surrounding light. Unfortunately, we noticed very soon the difficulty to use this cap. It makes the SoproCare bigger, and it is more difficult or even impossible to film some areas. We could not obtain a good image because a correct distance to the teeth is very important to have a good image and detect caries. We decided to do the research without the silicon cap. The surrounding light may have influenced our results.

An instrument to hold the mouth and cheeks open would theoretically also be better. We noticed soon that this only bothered the filming. Besides it was not pleasant for the inhabitants.

Secondly the filming was sometimes very time-consuming. With many teeth present, filming needed a lot more time than visual examination. Some elderly had problems with the duration because they were impatient or could not keep their mouth open if needed.

The filming was not as easy as it seemed. We constantly had to look at the computer screen during the filming to adjust our aim. The simplest and least time-consuming method was one examiner to film and a second to give instructions about how to move the camera and start/stop filming.

A video-making protocol was made before the start of our research. Very soon we noticed the difficulties of following this rule. Depending on the number and location of teeth, we modified our filming methods. It takes a lot more time to make 24 videos instead of, for example, 6, when some quadrants are filmed together. Sometimes we switched from one mode into another without interrupting the video. We individually estimated the most efficient way of filming.

6.4.2 Processing and Results

After these two examinations, we started interpreting the movies. Luckily, we gave every file a note with the location in the mouth during filming. This is very important considering orientation is lost as you cannot see surrounding structures on the videos. Caregivers in nursing homes will also be obliged to do so. This implicates to work with two or interrupt the examination after each movie to name it.

While interpreting the movies, we noticed that dentine is marked as red as caries due to the presence of porphyrins. This implicates no difference between an image of a teeth with attrition or one with incisal caries. Considering the importance to differentiate these two, we remarked a great disadvantage of the camera. On the other hand, interdental caries was strongly underdiagnosed.

Our results are processed using statistical methods presuming a normal distribution of data. To be certain of the results, more statistical calculations need to be done. We did not have enough statistical knowledge to do this, but a statistician will do it later.

Our examination loses its usefulness and preventive strength when patients are only interested in solving pain in their mouth. With a lot of elderly with orofacial problems, it was difficult to convince them to make a dentistry appointment.

6.5 Conclusion and Future Work

We can conclude that for less mobile elderly, it may be a relief that the necessity to go the dentist for their annual checkup is gone. The caregiver can scan the mouth and send the videos to the dentist who will interpret them. Thereby the calculus will not be removed, and the patients probably have no intention to go to the dentist only for cleaning. The soft tissues are scanned as well but the chance to miss something is not negligible. Considering a serious under diagnosis, it is possible that the dentist says that based on the videos everything is good, but a clinical oral examination would still reveal some problems. The SoproCare camera has a lot of good qualities, but we were not entirely convinced to use it for a consultation on distance.

Not only our working method can be ameliorated but also the habits and attitudes of the inhabitants. Obviously, we cannot help people who do not want to be helped or do not listen to our advice.

The attitude of dentists toward helping elderly in nursing homes can be better too. Only a very small number of dentist are prepared to go to nursing homes.

We cannot emphasize enough the need of preventive care regarding frail elderly. Further investigation is needed to explore the teledentistry system and his applicability in nursing homes. The other diagnostic tools as discussed previous can be tested as well. Maybe other diagnostic tools will be developed in the future.

References

1. De Visschere L, Janssens B, De Reu G, Duyck J, Vanobbergen J. An oral health survey of vulnerable older people in Belgium. Clin Oral Investig. 2015;20(8):1903–12.
2. De Visschere L, Vanobbergen J. Oral health care for frail elderly people: actual state and opinions of dentists towards a well-organised community approach. Gerodontologie. 2006;23:170–6.
3. WHO. World Oral Health Report. 2003. http://www.who.int/oral_health/publications/report03/en/.
4. Vanoverloop J, De Boeck T. Tandzorg bij ouderen in woonzorgcentra. s.l.: Studie voor Bond Moyson; 2007.
5. Luz PB, Stringhini DH, Otto BR, Port ALF, Zaleski V, Oliveira RS, Lussi A. Performance of undergraduate dental students on ICDAS clinical caries detection after different learning stages. Eur J Dent Educ. 2014;19:235–41.
6. International caries detection and assessment system. www.icdas.org: s.n.

7. Neeraj G, Pandit IK, Srivastava N, Gupta M, Sharma M. International Caries Detection and Assessment System (ICDAS): a new concept. Int J Clin Pediatr Dent. 2011;4(2):93–100.
8. Matthijs S, Moradi Sabzevar M, Adriaens PA. Intra-examiner reproducibility of 4 dental plaque indices. J Clin Periodontol. 2001;28(3):250–4.
9. Rechmann P, Liou SW, Rechmann BM, Featherstone JD. Performance of a light fluorescence device for the detection of microbial plaque and gingival inflammation. Clin Oral Investig. 2016;20(1):151–9.

e-Implantology

7

Dimitri Pascual and Vaysse Jérôme

Abstract

Introduction: Thanks to the digitalization of health data and thanks to computer-assisted implant surgery protocols, e-health enables a revolutionary exchange among experts on the topic. Thus it translates into an improvement of the quality of prosthetic rehabilitation on implants.

Technical Procedure: The overall data available for prosthetic rehabilitation on implants are now digital, reliable, and usable. Various experts on prosthetic rehabilitation can make use of a common software interface to validate the final prosthetic project before surgery and from a pluridisciplinary perspective. The software integrates the bone image, mucosal contours, dental imprint, occlusion, and facial scanner of the patient. Surgeon, dentist, prosthetist, and patient accept the surgical, occlusal, aesthetic, and conception constraints. The development of planning templates and guided surgical techniques allows a very precise virtual 3D modeling on the patient.

Discussion: Telemedicine and teleexpertise improve the quality, the security, the offer, and the access to implantology. New continuous digital workflow protocols remain without interruption. All the contributors decide and act to validate implant planning. This optimizes the prosthetic, occlusal, and aesthetic project, and it takes into account the surgical and bony constraints. Potential complications are clearly explained to the patient before surgery so that it is no longer an issue which will have to be justified postsurgery. Hence, the patient is completely

D. Pascual (✉)
Maxillo-facial Surgeon, Private Practice, 5 BD d'Estourmel, 12000 Rodez, France
e-mail: Dr.pascualdimitri@gmail.com

V. Jérôme
Dental Technician, 12 rue Falguière, 31000 Toulouse, France
e-mail: Contact@laboratoirehtd.com

N. Giraudeau (ed.), *e-Health Care in Dentistry and Oral Medicine*,
https://doi.org/10.1007/978-3-319-69450-4_7

satisfied when the temporary prosthesis is placed immediately. The implant surgery is simplified and therefore less stressful for both patient and surgeon. 3D planning with a numerical streaming component is indeed a pedagogical and communicative tool between surgeon, dentist, prosthetist, and patient.

Thanks to this exchange opportunity and to the collegial validation of a computer-assisted numerical streaming surgery, telemedicine and teleexpertise are in the process of becoming the technical choices to optimize accuracy and implant rehabilitation efficiency.

Keywords
Immediate dental implant loading • Dental implant-abutment design • Computer-assisted surgery • Image-guided surgery • Telemedicine

7.1 Introduction

The aesthetics and functionality of a prosthetics on an implant depend on the various bone, occlusal, prosthetic, and surgical constraints. The general health data that prosthetic rehabilitation on an implant requires are now digital, reliable, and ready for use. The digitalization of health data paired with computer-assisted implant surgery protocols enable a revolutionary exchange among experts on the topic. Through telemedicine and teleexpertise, e-health improves the offer, the quality, the security, and the access to this multidisciplinary implantology. Digital streaming enables all experts/contributors to determine and validate which is the ideal implant placement in the prosthetic project.

7.2 Technical Note

Practionners involved in the project use the coDiagnostiX® software (developed by Dental-wings® and Straumann®) as a platform to exchange data (Fig. 7.1). This numerical interface also serves as the prosthetic, the implant, and the making of a surgical guide planner.

First of all, a 3D maxillo-mandibular bone image must be formatted using DICOM (dental scanner or cone beam) and integrated into coDiagnostiX®. This image is matched with a digital dental imprint in the STL format (an intraoral camera or a regular one takes it and then a lab scanner digitalizes it). STL et DICOM digital files may be superimposed thanks to an easy identification of dental marks (sulcus in tooth, cuspid) (Fig. 7.2). In cases of partial or full edentulism, a bite block with radiopaque elements is placed in the mouth of the patient when the procuring of dental scanner takes place. These elements ensure an accurate repositioning of the dental and the gum imprint on the dental scanner (Fig. 7.3).

The surgeon or dentist then sends the mucosal and bone image file to the prosthetist lab via the software. The prosthetist models the prosthesis according to the dentist's request. He also takes into account the amount of prosthetic space, the gingival height,

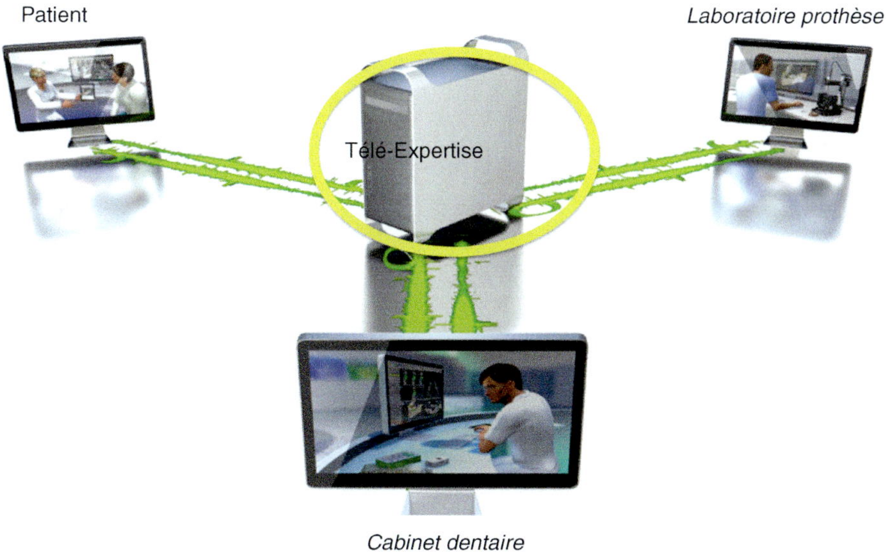

Fig. 7.1 Dataflow between teleexperts

Fig. 7.2 Digital overlay of DICOM (blue) and STL (yellow) file

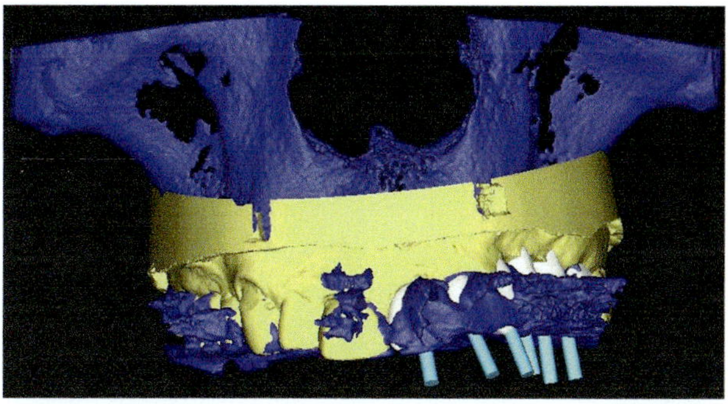

Fig. 7.3 Wax bite with radiopaque marker for the edentulous patient

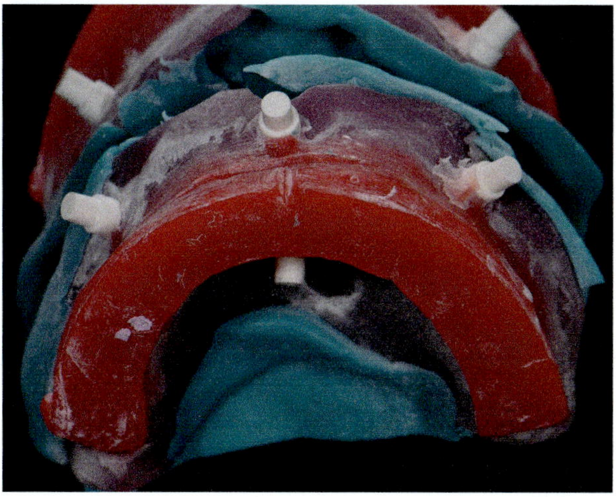

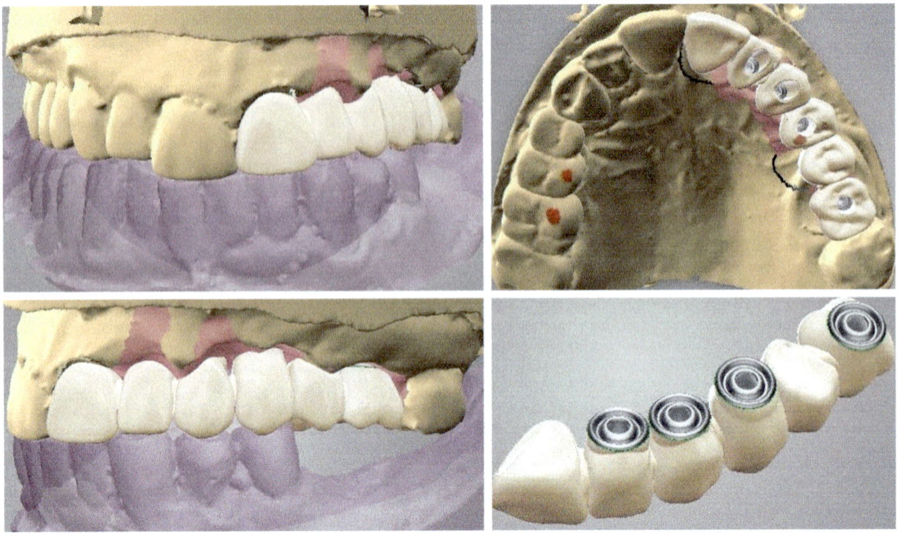

Fig. 7.4 Modeling the future prosthesis

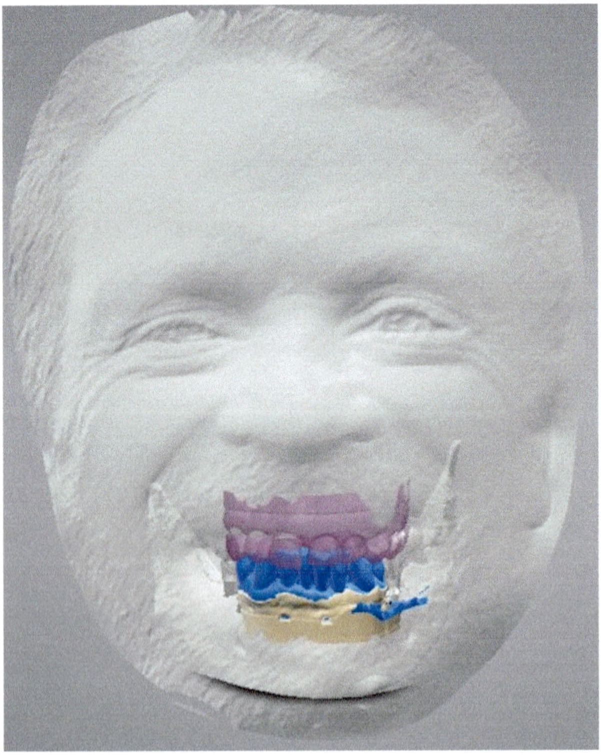

Fig. 7.5 Facial scanner

and mutually adjacent and antagonist teeth (Fig. 7.4). This file can be accompanied by a facial scanner to supply the aesthetic elements necessary to make the prosthetics such as facial symmetry and positioning and support of the lip at rest and smile (Fig. 7.5).

The new bone/mucosal/prosthesis file is sent back to the dentist so he may validate the prosthetic design; it is then forwarded to the surgeon so that he is able to virtually install the implants. The implant position and length depend on volume, density and bone quality, gingival height, tooth implant and implant-implant distances, implant parallelism, axis, and type of the future prothesis. The crown modeled on the software will therefore serve as a guide to the future implant axis and not the other way around (Fig. 7.6).

If for anatomical or surgical reasons the surgeon is unable to install the implants with the given prosthesis, he submits a new treatment plan to both dentist and prosthetist. This plan includes a compromise between the available bone volume, the keratinized gum, and the prosthetics. Multiple proposals may be exchanged until all parties come to a consensus and validate it all.

The software requires a copy of the original file before any modification is made. This allows for a traceability of all modifications so the practitioner can go back, if he wishes, to a previous modification.

Once the surgeon validates the new file, it is then transferred to the prosthetist so he is able to model the prosthetic pillar in accordance with the implant axis, the gum height, and the type of prosthetics.

Once the surgeon, the dentist, and the prosthetist validate the digital prosthetics and the implant position, the prosthetist makes a model of the surgical

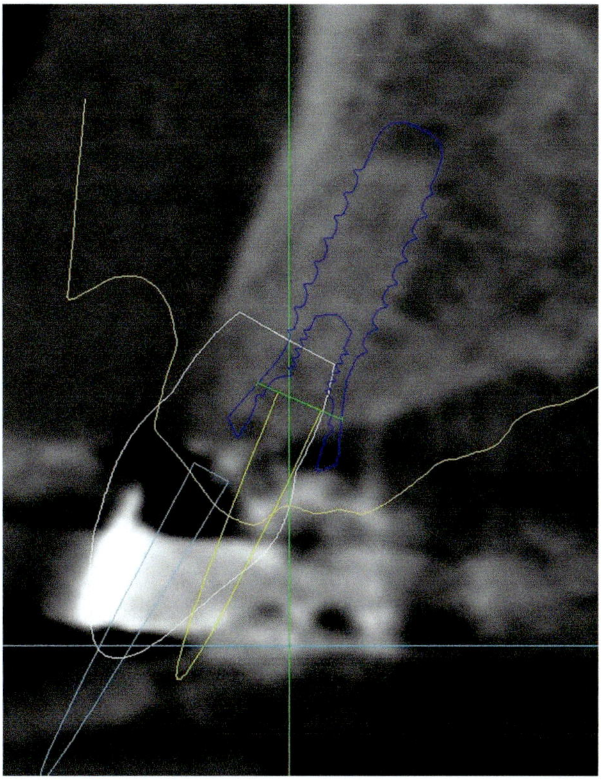

Fig. 7.6 Prosthesis as a guide for implant placement

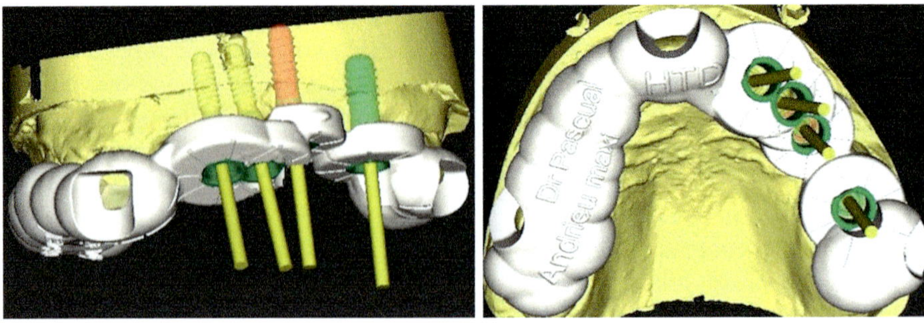

Fig. 7.7 Design guide

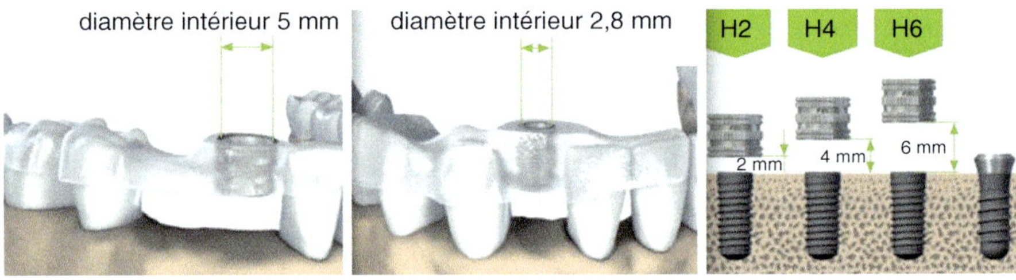

Fig. 7.8 Positioning of the drill bushings

guide (Fig. 7.7). He places a drilling bushing taking into account the gum height, the position of the tooth to be replaced, and the type and length of the implant. It serves as a guide for the implant axis, and it is a reference point regarding the height as the different steps of the drilling take place (Fig. 7.8).

Once all the experts have agreed to the implant planning, the surgical guide, and the prosthetics, the making of the implant may start.

The model for the arches, the temporary prosthesis, and the guide are made simultaneously. Guide and models are imprinted. The prosthesis is machined. The metallic bushings are secondarily inserted in the guide and fixated by friction.

In specialized centers, the machined prosthesis is secondarily adapted to a dental arch model with the exact position of the implants (Fig. 7.9). Before surgery, in the lab, the prosthetist makes adhere the resin to the titanium T-base. The prosthetist then perfects the occlusal contact points and the aesthetic aspect of the prosthesis.

The software determines the surgical protocol to follow with the various drilling sequences once the implant planning has been validated by all the experts (Fig. 7.10). The Straumann® surgical-guided case allows for a reproduction of all virtual implants positioning on the patient.

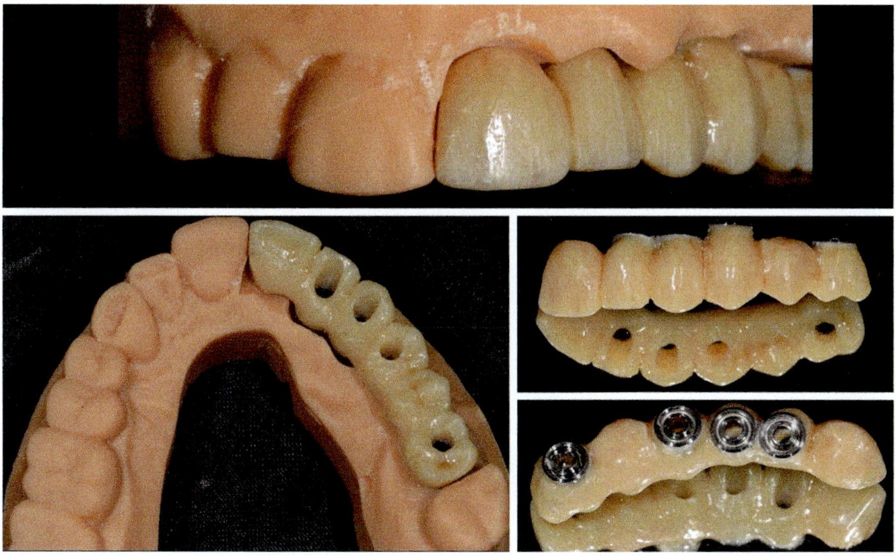

Fig. 7.9 Dental model and temporary prosthesis machined

Copie de CAB 2 guide2 — Protocole chirurgical — Système de la FDI (Fédération Dentaire Internationale)

Douille Straumann®Guided Surgery

Code couleur	Position	Réf. implant	Implant	Douille	Position de la douille	Foret guidé	Poignée de perçage	Fraise
	22	043.262S	Standard Plus Roxolid® SLA® (RN) Ø 3.3 mm 12 mm	H: 5 mm Ø: 5 mm	H4	≡ extra-long	●●● +3 mm	2.8 mm
	23	043.262S	Standard Plus Roxolid® SLA® (RN) Ø 3.3 mm 12 mm	H: 5 mm Ø: 5 mm	H4	≡ extra-long	●●● +3 mm	2.8 mm
	24	043.164S	Standard Plus Roxolid® SLA® (RN) Ø 4.1 mm 12 mm	H: 5 mm Ø: 5 mm	H2	= long	● +1 mm	3.5 mm
	26	043.068S	Standard Plus Roxolid® SLA® (RN) Ø 4.8 mm 10 mm	H: 5 mm Ø: 5 mm	H2	= long	●●● +3 mm	4.2 mm

Fig. 7.10 Surgical protocol

Dental and/or mucosal and/or bone and osteosynthesis abutments follow the surgical guide positioning (Fig. 7.11). When placing implants, the guided implant bearing has the same diameter than the bushing, leaving no room for any angulation or placement. The four cardinal points that are visible on the abutment are lined up with those of the guide, and they serve as an indication whether the connection between implant and pillar is perfectly connected. The single or multiple temporary prosthesis which has been modeled from the planning and made presurgery is immediately placed after the implants are put in (Figs. 7.12 and 7.13).

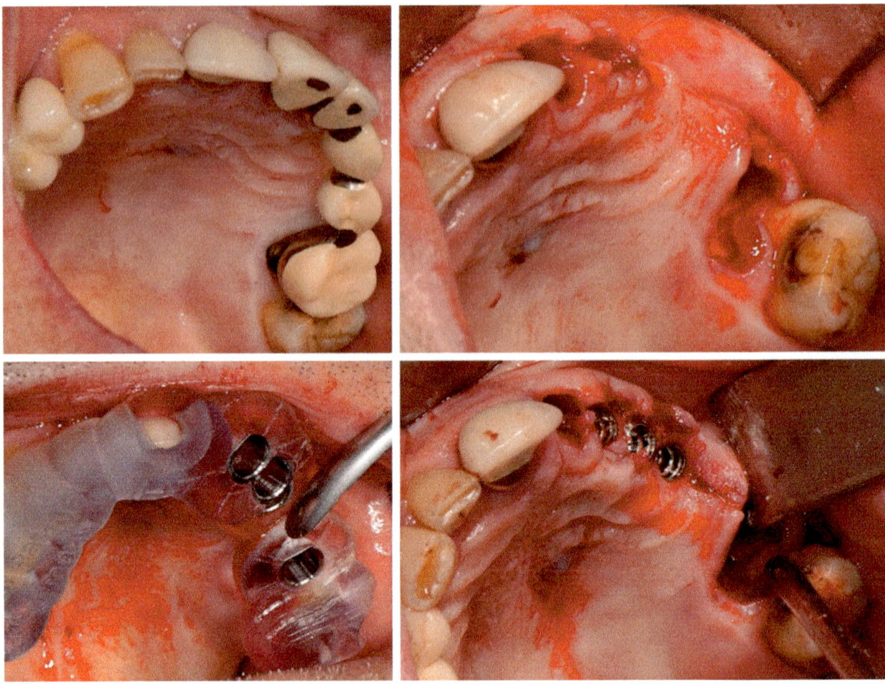

Fig. 7.11 Guided surgery

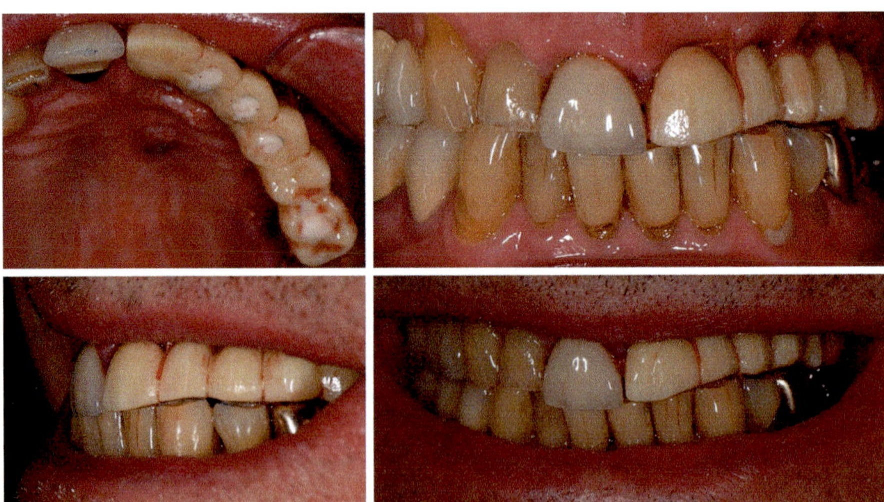

Fig. 7.12 Immediate loading of the prosthesis

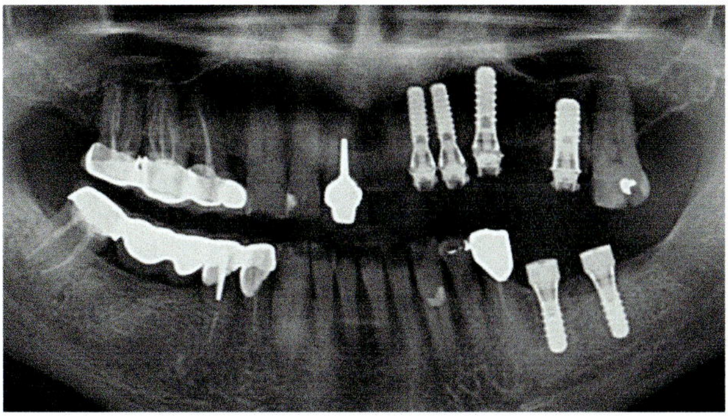

Fig. 7.13 Dental panoramic X-ray control

7.3 Discussion

E-health enables a revolutionary health exchange among expert practioners from different competencies and medical backgrounds.

Dental implant rehabilitation is complex, demanding, and costly for the patient. Surgeons, dentists, and prosthetists must be highly trained, and each must have access to technical expertise in the subject matter. Telemedicine allows a patient who lives in an isolated zone to ask for an expert opinion from a distance. This virtual care gives patients a new communicative and informational tool.

Many dentists can feel isolated when they are faced with offering implant options to their patients or simply if they need to follow up on their surgery. The regular dentist can assess if an implant is a viable option (via a clinical exam, X-rays, and digital imprint). A specialist can then give his expert opinion at a distance which is thorough, prompt, and satisfying for the patient. The expert consult is only needed if there is a doubt or for the surgery. It allows for a better time management between consultations and implant placement. The patient saves a great deal of unnecessary appointments. This optimizes implant possibilities for the patient, and it makes postsurgical follow-ups easier as well. Through exchanges, teleexpertise enables an efficient and pluridisciplinary care. It maximizes the quality and the security of the implant project.

Digital streaming improves the implant positioning as it reproduces the ideal position of the implant, first validated by the expert contributors in the prosthetic project [1–3]. New protocols have a continuous digital work flow: dental scanner (Dicom), imprint (STL), superposition of the dental scanner and the imprint, facial scanner, planning, printing of the surgical guide and the dental arch, milling of the temporary and the permanent prosthesis. There are currently other computer-assisted surgical aid software that do not offer a digital streaming component. A stone model has to be fabricated which diminishes accuracy.

Thanks to the software, surgeons, dentists, and prosthetists have total freedom to make the prosthesis and the guide or to position implants. They simply use a modifiable "open STL" file. They no longer depend on a guide maker who used to choose it all from guide to implant positioning. This resulted in problems when the permanent prosthesis was made. Now practitioners have total control over the final product.

Guided and computer-assisted surgery allows for a presurgical product making and validation. There is little to no gum flap detachment thanks to the mucosal incision [4]. The drill bushing handle is stabilized inside the drill tip. There is no risk for the drill.

The risk of drill impact point displacement by sliding during drilling an asymmetrical or protruding bone crest is absent. The primary stability of the implant is enhanced by a safe and quick drill passage which limits the risk of bone heating and roundness of drilling. The implant burying mark on the implant holder allows to place the apex of the implant precisely in contact with the downhole. The risk of grinding a peri-implant soft bone, upon rotation of the implant turns abutted in downhole, is absent. The implant axis control and the operating X-rays are not necessary. The operating time is reduced. Surgery is less invasive. The postoperative is simple. Prosthetic failures and collateral damage (nerve and adjacent root damage, intra-sinus implant, implant axis unusable) are avoided. Prosthetic project, occlusion and aesthetic, taking into account the bone and surgical constraints, is the most optimal as possible [1–3]. The immediate implementation of the provisory prosthesis ensures rapid patient satisfaction [5]. The implant surgery is simplified and less "stressful" for the patient and the surgeon [6, 7].

3D planning serves as an educational and communication tool between surgeon, prosthetist, dentist, and patient. It facilitates exchange and understanding about the prosthetic project. The visualization of the future crown before surgery allows to validate or modify the project, in a multidisciplinary way, to respect the patient's needs and the prosthetist, dentist, and surgeon constraints. The practitioner, knowing before the intervention ordre des mots pour meilleuresyntaxe: knowing the future implant position and the pillar type to use, can accurately inform the patient of the future prosthetic cost.

Conclusion

The anticipation of all risk factors have to be considered ahead of the surgery for limit the risk of failure in the prosthetic implant project. Surgical risks and errors man-made are minimized. All actors become actors-makers to validate the planning. The difficulties encountered in the project are explained to patients before surgery and no longer suffered or to be justified after surgery.

This technique is not to put in the hands of a beginner. Surgical and digital global vision is essential. Planning requires much attention and time. Planning errors are found during the surgery, and the technical difficulties are the same as for freehand surgery. It is necessary to have a good surgical implant experience to be able to manage the unexpected.

Telemedicine and teleexpertise, thanks to the possibility of exchange and collegial validation of guided and computer-assisted surgery in a continuous digital workflow, are becoming the choice of technical conditions to optimize the accuracy and efficiency of implant rehabilitation but require a learning curve, collaboration, and precise tuning between the surgeon, the dentist, the prosthetist, and the patient.

Thanks to the prosthetist Jerome Vaysse for the iconography and the quality of prosthetic achievements.

Conflict of Interest No conflict of interest.

References

1. Hämmerle CH, Stone P, Jung RE, Kapos T, Brodala N. Consensus statements and recommended clinical procedures regarding computer-assisted implant dentistry. Int J Oral Maxillofac Implants. 2009;24:126–31.
2. Ersoy AE, Turkyilmaz I, Ozan O, McGlumphy EA. Reliability of implant placement with stereolithographic surgical guides generated from computer tomography clinical data from 94 implants. J Periodontol. 2008;79:1339–45.
3. Davarpanah K, Demurashvili G, Daas M, Rajzbaum P, Capelle-Ouadah N, Szmukler-Moncler S, Davarpanah M. Implantologie assistée par ordinateur. Rev Stomatol Chir Maxillofac. 2012;113:335–49.
4. Moraschini V, Velloso G, Luz D, Porto Barboza E. Implant survival rates, marginal bone level changes, and complications in full-mouth rehabilitation with flapless computer-guided surgery: a systematic review and meta-analysis. Int J Oral Maxillofac Surg. 2015;44:892–901.
5. Stapleton BM, Lin WS, Ntounis A, Harris BT, Morton D. Application of digital diagnostic impression, virtual planning, and computer-guided implant surgery for a CAD/CAM-fabricated, implant-supported fixed dental prosthesis. J Prosthet Dent. 2014;112:402–8.
6. Sarment DP, Surkovic P, Clinthorne N. Accuracy of implant placement with a stereolithographic surgical guide. Int J Oral Maxillofac Implants. 2003;18:571–7.
7. Nickenig HJ, Wichmann M, Hamel J, Schlegel KA, Eitner S. Evaluation of the difference in accuracy between implant placement by virtual planning data and surgical guide templates versus the conventional free-hand method – a combined in vivo-in vitro technique using cone-beam CT (part II). J Craniomaxillofac Surg. 2010;38:488–93.

Teledentistry and Orthodontics

8

Murilo Fernando Neuppmann Feres, Maurilo de Mello Lemos, Marina Guimarães Roscoe, and Nicolas Giraudeau

Abstract

Teledentistry can be considered as a valuable tool to assist isolated or disadvantaged populations and to improve access to oral healthcare. The application of teledentistry has demonstrated interesting results in many fields of Dentistry. The objective of this chapter is to review the literature on the attempt to associate teledentistry and orthodontics. Most of the collected studies described and evaluated teledentistry as a means to improve effectiveness of orthodontic referrals and consultancy. Other researches focused on evaluating the use of teledentistry for remote diagnosis, monitoring, and motivation of orthodontic patients. After critically reviewing the collected evidence, it was considered that teledentistry might be used as a helpful tool for referring patients or providing consultancy to general practitioners. The possible benefits included the ability of decreasing the number of inappropriate referrals and encouraging previously trained general practitioners to treat cases. Minor issues, such as the small likelihood of patients being neglected, as well as the lack of standardization during records preparation, are still a concern. There is a clear trend among professionals toward a supportive position of teledentistry use allied with orthodontic practice. Nevertheless, most of the general practitioners still present concerns in relation to workload increase. Literature is still scarce on cost studies of teledentistry. It is therefore suggested that future researchers address that gap in addition to conduct methodologically stronger studies focused not only on the financial aspects of teledentistry, but also on the clinical outcomes of the treatment provided with the aid of this system.

Keywords

Teledentistry • Orthodontics • E-health care

M.F.N. Feres (✉) • M. de Mello Lemos • M.G. Roscoe
Guarulhos University, Guarulhos, Brazil
e-mail: murilo.feres@ung.br; mlemos@prof.ung.br; marina.roscoe@prof.ung.br

N. Giraudeau
University of Montpellier, Montpellier, France
e-mail: nicolas.giraudeau@umontpellier.fr

N. Giraudeau (ed.), *e-Health Care in Dentistry and Oral Medicine*,
https://doi.org/10.1007/978-3-319-69450-4_8

8.1 Introduction

In general terms, teledentistry (TD) is defined as the use of information technology and telecommunications for dental care, consultation, education, and public awareness [1]. It can be a valuable tool to assist isolated and disadvantaged populations that have limited access to specialized dental care [1, 2]. TD has the possibility of improving access to oral healthcare and lowering its costs. It also has the potential to eliminate the disparities in oral healthcare between rural and urban communities [3].

The application of TD has already produced interesting results in many dental fields [4]. The objective of this chapter is to bring the literature on the attempt to associate TD and orthodontics. Specifically, our objective is to report the studies on orthodontic referrals and consultancy taking place in public healthcare settings, as well as to mention researches on the use of TD for remote diagnosis, monitoring, and motivation of orthodontic patients. Throughout this chapter, we intend not only to present the successful results that have been documented so far, but also to mention the points that still require closer attention from researchers and healthcare providers. By means of a comprehensive review of the literature, we also aimed at suggesting future researches to address non-contemplated topics, in addition to indicating directions that might potentially motivate stakeholders toward TD uptake and possibly consolidate its use in the orthodontic healthcare area.

8.2 Referrals and Consultancy

One of the primary objectives of TD is to support the use of technologies to diagnose and provide advice about treatment over a distance [5]. That is precisely one of the most studied uses of TD in orthodontics, *i.e.*, referring patients from basic to specialized care and providing orthodontic remote consultancy to general dental practitioners (GDPs) [2, 6–8].

Almost all of the studies that will be presented in this section were sited in the United Kingdom (UK), where the orthodontic treatment for children is mostly covered by the National Health Service (NHS) [8]. Since there is reportedly unequal distribution of orthodontic specialists in the UK territory [9], GDPs are entitled to conduct less complex orthodontic treatments, considering individual levels of orthodontic skills.

Traditionally, NHS general practitioners customarily used letters to refer patients when they were either unsure whether it was a suitable case for them to treat, when they were sure they wanted to treat but needed advice about how to proceed, or when they were unsure about the referral/treatment timing [8]. Due to the absence of specific guidelines, referral patterns were reportedly excessive and, as a consequence, waiting lists tended to grow increasingly longer [10, 11]. With the implementation of the TD system, UK researchers [2, 6–8] sought to decrease waiting lists and to improve the speed of the referral procedures. Through the TD system, GDPs use technologies to send photographs, radiographs, and other important clinical information to orthodontists, in addition to participating in live video-conferences, by which direct communication with the orthodontist consultant is enabled.

Stephens et al. [8] firstly described the TD orthodontic referral/consultancy system as performed in a project sited in the University of Bristol, in England. In this trial, the authors recruited seven GDPs and one orthodontic consultant. Dentists had their practice fully equipped and were then submitted to training sessions on the use of the TD system. After carrying out a short-term trial, it was observed that inappropriate referral rates, due to poor timing, were reduced (approximately, 20%). This means that cases that would have been normally referred by conventional means actually were not, due to the advice remotely provided by the consultant. Furthermore, in nearly one-third of the cases, advices helped the practitioners to provide, by themselves, orthodontic treatment to children that would have been, otherwise, referred.

The results reported by these authors [8], although encouraging, were derived from a small sample and uncontrolled study, and therefore requires cautious interpretations. Hence, a longer-term prospective randomized study was posteriorly published [7] in order to evaluate the validity of a TD system for screening patients in a larger sample. In this instance, 15 Manchester dental practices were enrolled and were divided into two groups. The first one comprised of GDPs that would refer patients to orthodontic service via store-and-forward system, as the one we have just described [8]. Those referrals were compared to the ones made conventionally by other dental practices. Orthodontists would then receive referrals, through both means, and classify them as "accepted" or "not accepted". Professionals from both groups referred the same patients, and the classification obtained by direct observation was considered to be the gold standard.

There was moderate agreement of orthodontist acceptance rates of TD referrals. However, TD group was less likely to refer an individual who did not need orthodontic care than those who made referrals based on clinical examinations. Sensitivity of the TD system was 0.80 and specificity was 0.73. This means that the ability of the orthodontists to correctly identify proper/improper referrals, by means of TD system, is appropriate. However, there is still a risk of TD referrals being neglected, which would normally be accepted if referred by conventional means (approximately, 20%). This highlights a potential flaw in the validity or accuracy of TD to screen orthodontic referrals.

Mandall [6] had already published his first results on the reliability of photographs before his main manuscript, the one we have just described [12]. In this preliminary report [6], the researcher solely focused on reliability, and no comparisons with the conventional referral system were performed. There were relevant findings that, somehow, reinforce current recommendations for standardization of records, since interobserver agreement was considered low. Still, intra-examiner reliability was good, and it seemed to improve along the research period of time. In addition to standardization of records, this latter finding indicates the need for an adaptation period for the practitioners to get familiar with the TD system before actually referring patients for orthodontic advice.

Considering that orthodontic distance learning, in association with its technologies, has been successfully implemented in undergraduate and orthodontics programs over the past 15 years [13–18], it is our hope that TD will find, in the future, welcoming users that are theoretically more willing to implement technology as part of their work routine.

In the United States, Berndt et al. [2] conducted a research in Toppenish and Seattle (both in Washington), which compared orthodontic outcomes from interceptive treatments performed by non-orthodontists supervised by a specialist using real-time TD with those from orthodontic residents supervised by specialists on-site. For the remotely assisted group, videoconference units were set up at each site, allowing the orthodontist to communicate in real time with the GDP and the patient at chairside. It enabled the orthodontist to screen patients; provide instruction on treatment planning, bracket placement, and band appliances; follow up on treatment; and answer questions from the dentist, parent, or patients about treatment progress. Pre- and posttreatment orthodontic models from patients treated by both groups of operators (GDPs and residents) were assessed for the level of improvement after treatment (Peer Assessment Rating—PAR) [19].

Both groups of patients significantly decreased their PAR index, which indicates occlusal improvement. However, there was slightly more improvement in the direct supervision (44.1%, on average), in relation to the TD group (35.6%, on average), although these differences were not statistically significant. The results of this study suggest that the interceptive orthodontic treatment provided by GDPs and remotely supervised by orthodontic specialists is a viable approach. It is important to highlight, however, that GDPs had been previously subjected to training in interceptive orthodontics in this research. This fact demonstrates that, in addition to specialized supervision, GDPs should be ideally trained *a priori*, so their treatment results might potentially reach acceptable quality levels.

The set of studies analyzed thus far [2, 6–8] generally demonstrated that TD should be implemented in public healthcare services, considering its potential benefits, such as decreasing the number of inappropriate referrals [7, 8] and increasing GDP confidence for treating simpler cases [8]. Both benefits could theoretically act on reducing referral waiting lists, targeting one of the researchers' main concerns (long waiting lists). In addition, remotely-assisted GDPs have proven to be technically able to perform simpler orthodontic therapeutic approaches, as long as they receive previous orthodontic basic training and long-distance assistance [2].

Even though TD has the potential to generate positive effects in healthcare systems, with insignificant decrease in the quality of the orthodontic treatment provided, some points seem too important to be overlooked. According to the literature we have reviewed, a relevant number of patients is likely to be neglected [7], and records seem still too variably collected and prepared, which might hinder the TD system reliability. Evidences have already suggested that picture records standardization is reasonably feasible [20], and sensitivity could hypothetically be raised if records were made in an accurate and standardized fashion.

The provision of assistance by remote consultants tends to be well received by both professionals and users. Cook et al. [21] collected GDPs' opinions on a remote orthodontic advice service. After four months of use, the general response to the TD system was very good. Among the positive replies, GDPs found that TD was a good way of getting advice, and it was particularly useful in borderline cases. Dentists were happy with the time length it took to get the advice. Patients and parents were particularly keen on the new system. As a downside, dentists were concerned about the additional time that preparing the cases, especially digital images, would probably take. Despite the extra-time consumption, none of the GDPs reported great difficulties with using the equipment to prepare cases, and the educational process was reported to be rewarding as well.

According to a previously reported research [8], sited in Bristol, most of the interviewed GDPs required technical support in the earlier stages of system use. All the dentists found that sending files was quite straightforward. Although live video links provided fast responses, it was not perceived as essential by GDPs. Videoconferences were rather useful from an educational point of view. In addition to all of those advantages, as perceived by GDPs, TD system was universally accepted by both patients and parents. But authors reported financial-related concerns, since additional time would be supposedly necessary for GDPs to prepare and send the cases.

Mandall et al. [12] have also evaluated Manchester GDPs' perception on TD for orthodontic referral purposes. Most of the GDPs were certain that professional communication and, as a consequence, guidance and advice would be enhanced with TD. However, they were not sure whether electronic referrals would actually help shorten waiting lists. Increased time in the surgery and incompatible remuneration were confirmed as potential concerns by most of the GDPs. According to reports, there were also concerns about equipment security and patient confidentiality and consent.

Bradley et al. [22] also investigated the opinions taken from GDPs of West Yorkshire regarding an online orthodontic referral service. Professionals were enquired into their orthodontic treatment and referral patterns, as well as into their attitudes to the use of the Internet and related technologies. As replies were collected, just under half of the respondents would be interested in using TD to obtain an orthodontist's advice, reasons being saving time and achieving fast opinions for treatment planning. However, a substantial number of GDPs remained undecided, possibly because they were unsure of their technology background. The reason of this result might be due to the fact that less than half of the respondents stated that they had access to Internet in their practices. Nearly 40% of the respondents perceived TD as helpful for patients.

Stephens and Cook [23] have otherwise collected the consultants' opinion on the remote counseling system. Nearly two hundred orthodontists answered a questionnaire on their functions and the system, as a whole. The minority opposed to the implementation of a national advice service. Most of the consultants were interested in providing an electronic diagnostic service for GDPs, and 70% were in favor of further research into providing advice by electronic means. However, the respondents still demonstrated concerns regarding medico-legal aspects, workload increase, quality of image records, and the suitability of their advice, once they would be unaware of each GDP's individual skills.

In spite of few inconsistencies [22], literature generally shows GDPs and consultants as supportive actors of TD for referring purposes [8, 12, 21, 23]. However, there are still minor issues that should be taken into consideration, such as additional time required to prepare cases and incompatible remuneration [8, 12, 21]. Additional concerns refer to security, confidentiality, and consent issues [12]. Once again, we emphasize the importance of training and the need of prior familiarization with the TD system by its users. In addition, softwares should be developed to make the preparation/sending records faster; and since GDPs might require further time and workload for having cases prepared and sent, it is also suggested monetary reimbursement as an incentive for TD uptake by GDPs.

8.3 Use of TD for Diagnosis and Patient Monitoring

There have been some descriptions in the literature for potentially useful purposes of technology for remote diagnosis and orthodontic patient monitoring [24–27].

One of the main difficulties encountered by clinicians refers to the application of reliable methods for soft tissue assessment [28]. Despite the important innovation brought by tridimensional examination modalities [28, 29], static records inherently present limitations in relation to the evaluation of orthodontic patients lip posture. Considering such a disadvantage, Zamzam and Luther [26] compared two methods of dynamic assessment of lip position in cerebral palsy and unaffected children. In their research, the authors evaluated the validity of a video surveillance system as an alternative means of obtaining reliable records of children in relation to their mouth resting posture (open or closed). The method under evaluation comprised of a video camera that recorded patients during their routine activities, which would allow unobtrusive observations from professionals. This assessment method was compared with clinical direct examination. Patients' lip position was classified [30], and the agreement rates between both methods were calculated. Even though intra-examiner agreement rates were just moderate for both methods individually, agreement between the remote surveillance system and the direct examination was considered to be good. This result implies that the video recording of patients might be considered an adequate tool for lip posture diagnosis. This method can be especially useful when it comes to the evaluation of children with suspected oral respiration, since open-mouth posture of mouth breathers has been proven to cause detrimental effects to craniofacial growth and occlusion development [31–33]. Furthermore, considering that orthodontic treatment success is dependent on patient cooperation, video recording could be also regarded as a virtually important tool to monitor patients' adherence to treatment. Video records could probably help clinicians dealing with noncooperative patients that would be benefited from video feedback as a means of increasing their adherence. After proper consent, such records should be preferably obtained in a standardized way, so reliable and reproducible data can be collected.

Orthodontic "difficult" cases, as characterized by orthodontists themselves, are most likely to be related to problems with oral hygiene, compliance, and patient request for more appointments [34]. Considering this scenario, minor orthodontic emergencies could also be solved from the use of this remote monitoring of patients. Favero et al. [24] equipped ten young orthodontic patients with a mobile videophone. They were asked to use their devices to contact the orthodontist for advice in case of minor emergencies, such as food impaction between teeth, ligature displacement, discomfort, lesions, irritation of lips and cheeks, displacement of the archwire, and bracket detachment or band debonding. During the whole period of their orthodontic treatment, most of the emergencies were easily addressed at home. In addition, the perceived level of satisfaction was high. Considering that remote assistance such as these can be easily delivered and that they proved to be effective, we see no objection on endorsing the use of this resource on private practices or public health services. That would certainly decrease the costs and disturbance for patients, professionals, or healthcare systems.

Zotti et al. [27] tested an app-based approach for oral hygiene maintenance in adolescents. Patients undergoing orthodontic treatment with full-fixed appliances were divided into two groups. Patients from the study group were enrolled in a WhatsApp group in which they were encouraged to make part of a competition and to share "selfies" showing their oral hygiene status. Pictures should be taken before and after using the plaque-disclosing tablets, and patients were ranked on a weekly basis taking into consideration their hygiene status. WhatsApp group users were allowed to interact with each other and to share information, pictures, and movies regarding oral hygiene and orthodontic treatment. After six months of treatment, the study group demonstrated better rates of plaque and gingival indices in comparison with the control group. After the ninth month of treatment, significantly lower incidences of white spot lesions and caries were observed for the study group.

Mupparapu [25], in his manuscript, strongly advocated the adoption of Voice over Internet Protocol (VoIP) technology, *e.g.*, Skype, in private practice offices as an alternative to regular telephone service. According to the author, VoIP can yield significant cost savings. It is more affordable than the traditional telephone service and can be easily installed in any office that has broadband connectivity.

In conclusion, it appears highly recommendable that such tools be implemented in orthodontic clinical practice, as a routine basis. At most of the times, technologies used to remotely monitor, diagnose, communicate to, and motivate patients are affordable and can bring relevant effects for both patients and practitioners. It seems evident, however, that all resources should be custom-tailored for each purpose, patient, and clinical environment, considering essential goals such as the patient oral health improvement, cost savings, and productivity increase. The most prominent concern from the patient perspective is the confidentiality of the data [4, 35]. Therefore, one should also keep in mind that any sort of privacy-related issues, as well as ethical and legal concerns, must necessarily be addressed before the implementation of any system.

8.4 Final Considerations

One of the most promising fields for TD implementation is certainly the public health, especially in countries of resource-constrained economies [36]. The availability and the application of such versatile resources in researches, as well as the innumerous possibilities they bring along, might certainly captivate potential users, patients, researchers, and health policy makers.

Concerning the orthodontics field, TD can be used as a helpful tool for referring patients or providing help to general practitioners during diagnosis, treatment planning, or even simpler therapeutic procedures [37]. It might be also useful in cases of minor emergency procedures, patient education, and motivation [37].

Conclusion

Several well-succeeded researches have demonstrated that TD might be useful, feasible, and highly likely to be accepted by its users. Nevertheless, there still seems to be just few researches dedicated to investigate TD cost-effectiveness. There is still need for more homogeneous and methodologically stronger studies examining clinical outcomes, healthcare utilization, and costs in greater depth, which are critical for evidence base [38]. TD is a fast-growing field with a lot of potential, but more emphasis needs to be put on allocation of funds and grants to conduct more clinical trials and to identify how TD can play a role in the provision of oral healthcare [39].

References

1. Clark GT. Teledentistry: what is it now, and what will it be tomorrow? J Calif Dent Assoc. 2000;28(2):121–7.
2. Berndt J, Leone P, King G. Using teledentistry to provide interceptive orthodontic services to disadvantaged children. Am J Orthod Dentofac Orthop. 2008;134(5):700–6.
3. Singh V, Bhaskar DJ, Chandan Agali R, Kishore M, Bumb S, Kadtane SS. Teledentistry: it's all about access to care. TMU J Dent. 2014;1(2):64–6.
4. Jampani ND. Applications of teledentistry: a literature review and update. J Int Soc Prev Community Dent. 2011;1(2):37–44.
5. Fricton J, Chen H. Using teledentistry to improve access to dental care for the underserved. Dent Clin N Am. 2009;53(3):537–48.
6. Mandall NA. Are photographic records reliable for orthodontic screening? J Orthod. 2002;29(2):125–7.
7. Mandall NA, O'Brien KD, Brady J, Worthington HV, Harvey L. Teledentistry for screening new patient orthodontic referrals. Part 1: a randomised controlled trial. Br Dent J. 2005;199(10):659–62.
8. Stephens C, Cook J, Mullings C. Orthodontic referrals via TeleDent Southwest. Dent Clin N Am. 2002;46(3):507–20.
9. Collins JM, Cunningham SJ, Moles DR, Galloway J, Hunt NP. Factors which influence working patterns of orthodontists in the United Kingdom. Br Dent J. 2009;207(1):E1.
10. O'Brien K, McComb JL, Fox N, Bearn D, Wright J. Do dentists refer orthodontic patients inappropriately? Br Dent J. 1996;181(4):132–6.

11. Rayner WJ, Neal JJ. Pre-assessment triage of orthodontic referrals at an East Yorkshire Hospital. Br Dent J. 2008;204(9):493–5.
12. Mandall NA, Qureshi U, Harvey L. Teledentistry for screening new patient orthodontic referrals. Part 2: GDP perception of the referral system. Br Dent J. 2005;199(11):727–9.
13. Al-Jewair TS, Azarpazhooh A, Suri S, Shah PS. Computer-assisted learning in orthodontic education: a systematic review and meta-analysis. J Dent Educ. 2009;73(6):730–9.
14. Brains M, Reynolds PA, McDonald F, Sherriff M. Effectiveness and acceptability of face-to-face, blended and e-learning: a randomised trial of orthodontic undergraduates. Eur J Dent Educ. 2011;15(2):110–7.
15. Komolpis R, Johnson RA. Web-based orthodontic instruction and assessment. J Dent Educ. 2002;66(5):650–8.
16. Miller KT, Hannum WM, Morley T, Proffit WR. Use of recorded interactive seminars in orthodontic distance education. Am J Orthod Dentofac Orthop. 2007;132(3):408–14.
17. Nurko C, Proffit WR. Acceptability and perceived effectiveness of web-based self-instruction in clinical orthodontics. Angle Orthod. 2005;75(4):521–5.
18. Shastry S, Park JH. Evaluation of the use of digital study models in postgraduate orthodontic programs in the United States and Canada. Angle Orthod. 2014;84(1):62–7.
19. Richmond S, Shaw WC, O'Brien KD, Buchanan IB, Jones R, Stephens CD, Roberts CT, Andrews M. The development of the PAR index (peer assessment rating): reliability and validity. Eur J Orthod. 1992;14(2):125–39.
20. Mok CW, Zhou L, McGrath C, Hägg U, Bendeus M. Digital images as an alternative to orthodontic casts in assessing malocclusion and orthodontic treatment need. Acta Odontol Scand. 2007;65(6):362–8.
21. Cook J, Edwards J, Mullings C, Stephens C. Dentists' opinions of an online orthodontic advice service. J Telemed Telecare. 2001;7(6):334–7.
22. Bradley SM, Williams S, D'Cruz J, Vania A. Profiling the interest of general dental practitioners in West Yorkshire in using teledentistry to obtain advice from orthodontic consultants. Prim Dent Care. 2007;14(3):117–22.
23. Stephens CD, Cook J. Attitudes of UK consultants to teledentistry as a means of providing orthodontic advice to dental practitioners and their patients. J Orthod. 2002;29(2):137–42.
24. Favero L, Pavan L, Arreghini A. Communication through telemedicine: home teleassistance in orthodontics. Eur J Paediatr Dent. 2009;10(4):163–7.
25. Mupparapu M. Voice over internet protocol for the orthodontic practice: a sensible switch from plain old telephone service. Am J Orthod Dentofac Orthop. 2008;133(3):470–5.
26. Zamzam N, Luther F. Comparison of lip incompetence by remote video surveillance and clinical observation in children with and without cerebral palsy. Eur J Orthod. 2001;23(1):75–84.
27. Zotti F, Dalessandri D, Salgarello S, Piancino M, Bonetti S, Visconti L, Paganelli C. Usefulness of an app in improving oral hygiene compliance in adolescent orthodontic patients. Angle Orthod. 2016;86(1):101–7.
28. Fourie Z, Damstra J, Gerrits PO, Ren Y. Accuracy and reliability of facial soft tissue depth measurements using cone beam computer tomography. Forensic Sci Int. 2010;199(1-3):9–14.
29. Metzger TE, Kula KS, Eckert GJ, Ghoneima AA. Orthodontic soft-tissue parameters: a comparison of cone-beam computed tomography and the 3dMD imaging system. Am J Orthod Dentofac Orthop. 2013;144(5):672–81.
30. Jackson D. Lip positions and incisor relationship. Brit Dent J. 1962;112(2):147–55.
31. Feres MF, Muniz TS, de Andrade SH, Lemos Mde M, Pignatari SS. Craniofacial skeletal pattern: is it really correlated with the degree of adenoid obstruction? Dental Press J Orthod. 2015;20(4):68–75.
32. Lessa FC, Enoki C, Feres MF, Valera FC, Lima WT, Matsumoto MA. Breathing mode influence in craniofacial development. Braz J Otorhinolaryngol. 2005;71(2):156–60.
33. Lione R, Buongiorno M, Franchi L, Cozza P. Evaluation of maxillary arch dimensions and palatal morphology in mouth-breathing children by using digital dental casts. Int J Pediatr Otorhinolaryngol. 2014;78(1):91–5.

34. Cassinelli AG, Firestone AR, Beck FM, Vig KW. Factors associated with orthodontists' assessment of difficulty. Am J Orthod Dentofac Orthop. 2003;123(5):497–502.
35. Sfikas PM. Teledentistry legal and regulatory issues explored. J Am Dent Assoc. 1997;128(12):1716–8.
36. Mathews MA, Kathavate RN, Tewary S, Pawashe K. Teledentistry: a new frontier. IJOCR. 2015;3(10):1–6.
37. Batham PR, Kalia UDP, Dilliwal S. Teledentistry and its role in orthodontic patient management. J Stomat Occ Med. 2014;7(1):6–12.
38. Daniel SJ, Wu L, Kumar S. Teledentistry: a systematic review of clinical outcomes, utilization and costs. J Dent Hyg. 2013;87(6):345–52.
39. Khan SA, Omar H. Teledentistry in practice: literature review. Telemed J E Health. 2013;19(7):565–7.

E-Health Care in Oral Cancer

9

Anaclàudia Pereira Costa Flores, Erno Harzheim, Manoela Domingues Martins, Marcelo Rodrigues Gonçalves, Marco Antonio Trevizani Martins, Michelle Roxo Gonçalves, Otávio Pereira D'Avila, Roberto Nunes Umpierre, and Vinicius Coelho Carrard

Abstract

Diagnosis of oral mucosal lesions, including oral cancer, is often challenging for the general dentists. This may be explained, at least in part, by the lack of training during undergraduate course. In this scenario, e-health initiatives have potential to help the health professionals, by means tele-education, teleconsulting, telediagnosis and interventions in the referral system to specialized consultations. This chapter summarizes the TelessaúdeRS/UFRGS actions to improve the quality of care in Oral Medicine in the Rio Grande do Sul State (Southern Brazil).

Keywords

Access to care • Health services research • Community dentistry • Decision-making

---

A.P.C. Flores • M.D. Martins • M.A.T. Martins • M.R. Gonçalves
Department of Oral Pathology, School of Dentistry,
Federal University of Rio Grande do Sul, Porto Alegre, Brazil

E. Harzheim
School of Medicine, Federal University of Rio Grande do Sul, Porto Alegre, Brazil

M.R. Gonçalves • R.N. Umpierre
School of Medicine, Federal University of Rio Grande do Sul, Porto Alegre, Brazil
TelessaúdeRS/UFRGS, Porto Alegre, Brazil

O.P. D'Avila (✉)
TelessaúdeRS/UFRGS, Porto Alegre, Brazil
e-mail: otaviopereiradavila@gmail.com

V.C. Carrard
Department of Oral Pathology, School of Dentistry,
Federal University of Rio Grande do Sul, Porto Alegre, Brazil
TelessaúdeRS/UFRGS, Porto Alegre, Brazil

N. Giraudeau (ed.), *e-Health Care in Dentistry and Oral Medicine*,
https://doi.org/10.1007/978-3-319-69450-4_9

9.1 Introduction

Oral cancer is among the most prevalent malignant lesions worldwide [1, 2]. The global incidence of lip, oral cavity, and pharyngeal cancer, which currently account for 3.8% of all cancer cases, is predicted to rise by 62%, to 856,000 cases, by 2035 [3]. Because of the associated high morbidity and mortality, oral cancer has become a major public health issue [4]. Despite the many studies performed to identify alternative treatments, not much progress has been made to improve the prospects of patients with squamous cell carcinoma (SCC), the most frequent type of oral cancer, whose mortality rate has remained stable at about 50% in the past decades [5].

Early diagnosis of SCC is facilitated by the position of the mouth, which favors direct visual examination, and also by the fact that SCC originates in the epithelial surface. Nevertheless, diagnosis is often delayed, leading to the need for more aggressive treatments with worse prognosis [6–8].

Of all health-care professionals, general dental practitioners are in a privileged position to identify potentially malignant oral lesions [7]. However, many professionals find it hard to detect, diagnose, and treat oral mucosal lesions [9]. This fact has been attributed to the little time dedicated to undergraduate or postgraduate training in oral medicine, with little opportunity for evaluating patients and performing biopsies [10–12]. As a result, professionals who find it difficult or who feel unprepared to diagnose and treat oral lesions tend to refer a high number of patients to specialists [13]. This contributes to low resolvability at the primary care level and generates a backlog of specialty consultations. Additionally, some referral systems face difficulties in classifying referrals on the basis of risk for malignancy, and thus more urgent cases are not prioritized. In daily practice, that means delay in diagnosis of cancer and other oral mucosal lesions.

In this context, the potential benefits of e-health initiatives in oral medicine seem evident. In Brazil, TelessaúdeRS/UFRGS (www.ufrgs.br/telessauders), a telehealth program sponsored by the national Ministry of Health and by the state government of Rio Grande do Sul, has since 2007 developed a series of tele-education, teleconsulting, and telediagnosis actions focusing on oral health. The program encompasses a large research effort aimed at designing and evaluating systemic solutions to overcome the challenge of fragmented health-care delivery in Rio Grande do Sul, the southernmost Brazilian state. The project is headquartered in Porto Alegre (state capital) and is supported by the Federal University of Rio Grande do Sul. The present chapter intends to depict the telehealth services in oral medicine developed by TelessaúdeRS/UFRGS for primary care professionals, summarizing the weaknesses and strengths of e-health initiatives in oral medicine, specifically teleconsulting, tele-education, and telediagnosis.

9.2 Teleconsulting

9.2.1 Description

TelessaúdeRS/UFRGS (TSRS) has provided teleconsulting support for primary health-care (PHC) professionals on oral health issues since 2007. Among the teleconsultations, a significant number is related to oral medicine, comprising theoretical questions, and also requests for case discussion to support decision-making in relation to diagnosis and management. Between 2009 and 2016, approximately 30% of the total requests in the period corresponded to oral medicine issues. For questions about theoretical aspects, consultants prepare a slide presentation (if real-time videoconsulting) or written materials (if asynchronous teleconsulting) about the topic. For "case discussions," consultants discuss the clinical case and go over differential diagnoses. Sometimes, complementary tests or clinical management steps are recommended. Depending on the quality of the clinical data, a diagnostic hypothesis is suggested. A protocol was designed to help consultants select the best databases (including Cochrane, Pubmed, Clinical Evidence) to be searched for evidence. Requesters have included dentists (88%), physicians (10%), and nurses (2%).

9.2.2 Types of Teleconsulting

Two types of teleconsulting are available to TSRS users for clarification of issues regarding oral medicine:

Asynchronous teleconsulting (*62.5%*): Requesters submit their questions via a web platform. The consultant receives the request in his/her mailbox and then prepares a written answer supported by the scientific literature within 72 h (Fig. 9.1).

Real-time videoconsulting (*37.5%*): Requester and consultant schedule a Skype chat to discuss specific topics or clinical cases. Figure 9.2 shows a video consultation on the topic "how to diagnose oral cancer?"

9.2.3 Cons

- *Non-standardized requests*: The information sent with the request is often lacking or vague, mainly in relation to specific clinical cases. In other words, saying that "an ulcer was observed on the border of the tongue," with no information regarding duration or presence of pain or without information about other irritants, makes diagnosis difficult. Sometimes, the consultant has to ask for more detailed data to ensure an accurate opinion.
- *Lack of clinical images*: The great majority of cases are not accompanied by images. Hence, the evaluation must rely only on a clinical description which, in general, is not sufficiently accurate.
- *Low usage*: Given the evidence showing that many dentists do not feel confident to evaluate oral lesions, it seems that the number of professionals using the service is far below the potential number of users that would profit from technical help.

9.2.4 Pros

- *Qualified support*: Any PHC physician or dentist has easy access to specialist opinion and high-level information.
- *Issues mapping*: Opportunity for identifying problems in the health-care system and, consequently, for proposing strategies to overcome them.

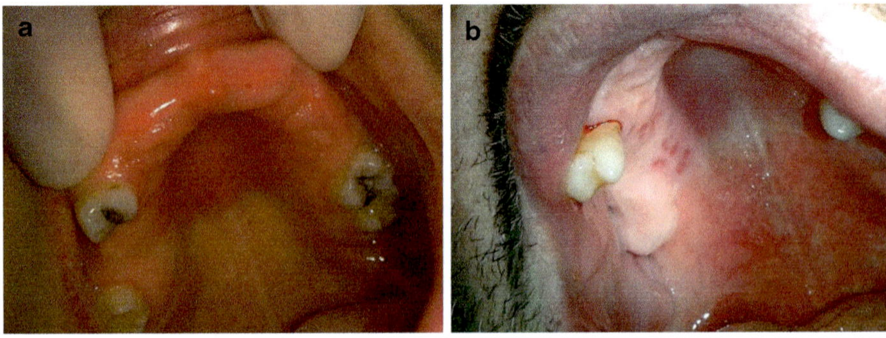

Case	Clinical data (Requester)	Response (Consultant)
A	35-year-old white female using removable dental prosthesis. Presents red lesion in hard palate, with rough surface, no symptoms. Clinical impression: denture-related stomatitis. I recommended removal of the prosthesis at night, and scheduled an appointment for 15 later. If there is no remission, what should I do? Biopsy? Refer to specialist? City: Vale do Sol/RS (183 km from Porto Alegre)	Diagnostic hypothesis: - Chronic atrophic candidiasis Management: - Nystatin oral suspension 100,000 IU/mL Oral rinse (3 minutes, 4 times/day, 14 days) - Removal and disinfection of prosthesis at night
B	52-year-old white male, smoker (20 cigarettes/day, 25 years), poor oral hygiene, no prosthesis. Lesion on alveolar ridge. Clinical impression: nicotinic stomatitis. City: Vale do Sol/RS (183 km from Porto Alegre)	Diagnostic hypothesis: - Secondary herpes infection Management: - Provide clinical advice and follow up

Fig. 9.1 (**a**, **b**) Clinical images and related data of cases discussed via asynchronous teleconsulting to support decision-making and confirm diagnosis

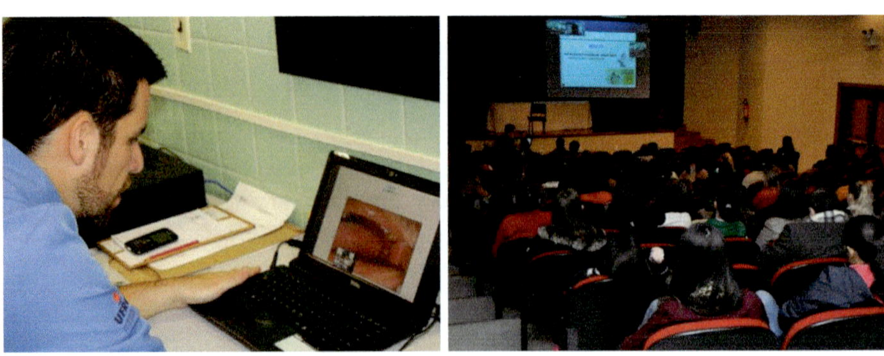

Fig. 9.2 Images of real-time videoconsulting with the specialist. The consultant is speaking from the School of Dentistry at the Federal University of Rio Grande do Sul, located in Porto Alegre (state capital) to an audience of about 70 people (dentists and undergraduate students) in Erechim, a municipality located 373 km away from Porto Alegre

9.3 Tele-education (2010–2017)

Few tele-education initiatives have been proposed in oral medicine worldwide [14]. The experience of TSRS with teleconsulting allowed the identification of knowledge gaps that we perceived as apt for educational interventions.

9.3.1 Webpalestra (Weblecture) (Fig. 9.3a, c, e)

Definition: Class focused on specific topics following a conventional lecture format. *Format*: Live lecture supported by slide presentation shared on-screen with the audience using a videoconferencing platform (WebConf—Adobe connect). The audience can chat, make comments, or send questions to presenters. The presentation is recorded and later made available on the TSRS website. Some weblectures were edited into shorter video podcasts that were uploaded to the TSRS YouTube channel and TSRS website.

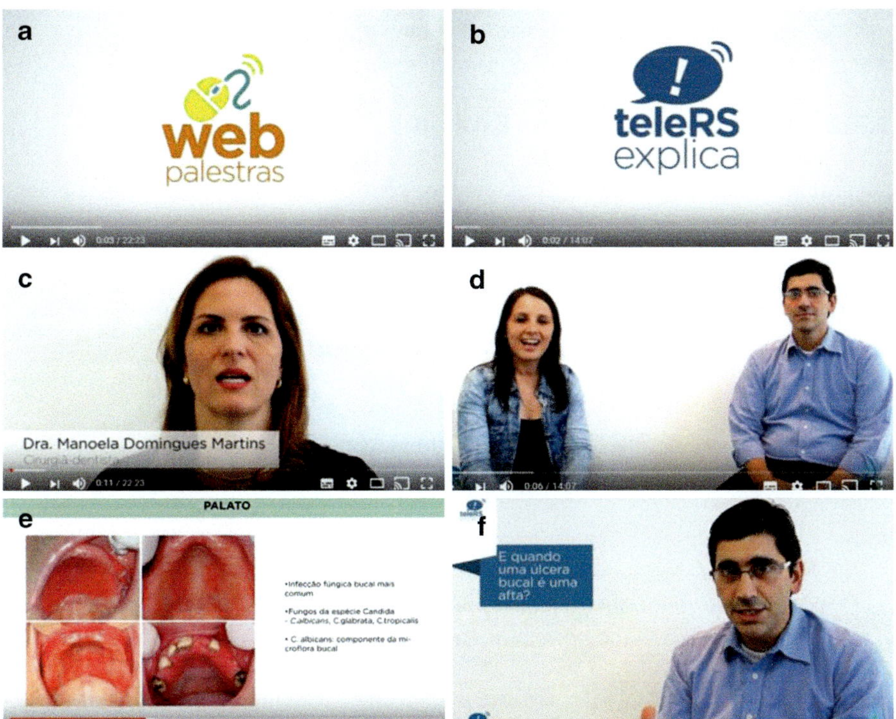

Fig. 9.3 Images of weblecture about erosive lesions presented by Professor Manoela Domingues Martins (**a**, **c**, **e**), and of the "TeleRS Explains" program entitled "Not every ulcer in your mouth is a cold sore," presented by (**b**, **d**, **f**) Professor Marco Antonio Trevizani Martins

Duration: 30–40 min.
Target audience: PHC professionals.
Topics

- Oral lesions (not available in YouTube).
- Oral cancer diagnosis in primary health care (6471 views).
- Differential diagnosis of white lesions of the oral cavity (not available in YouTube).
- Differential diagnosis of oral erosive lesions (490 views).
- Dental management of patients in current use of bisphosphonates (627 views).

Pros

- Knowledge spread to health-care professionals working at remote locations (in Rio Grande do Sul and other Brazilian States).
- Potential to increase awareness about oral lesions.

Cons

- Low audience.
- Low potential to change professional behavior.

9.3.2 TeleRS Explica (Telers Explains)

Definition: Interviews focusing on specific, controversial topics using a language that is accessible to the population in general.
Format: Short video made available in YouTube and TSRS website. This format does not allow interaction between presenters and audience.
Duration: 10–20 min.
Target audience: Health-care professionals and population in general.
Topics

- "Not every oral ulcer is a cold sore" (490 views).
- "Not all burning in the mouth is burning mouth syndrome" (1618 views).

Pros

- Opportunity to point out misconceptions regarding oral lesions.
- Opportunity to reach the population and increase the knowledge on oral health.

Cons

- Small audience.
- Lack of evidence of real impact.

9.3.3 E-Learning

Considering that specific educational interventions may have little impact on the knowledge and behavior of health-care professionals, we created an oral medicine training course. The proposed syllabi cover basic topics such as the evaluation process (see below) as well as different types of oral lesions. Since 2010, the program was offered five times; however, because the approach changed significantly from the first to the latest issue, two separate phases can be described:

9.3.3.1 Phase 1

Format

- Content-based instruction: lectures addressing detailed information on each lesion, grouping according to clinical type.
- Conventional lecture using slides with narration and case discussions based on slide presentations.
- Course made available in an institutional e-learning platform (Moodle UFRGS).

Duration: 20–26 h over 10 weeks.
Audience: Dentists, physician, nurses, and dieticians (maximum 62 participants).
Editions: Four (two in 2010, 2013, 2014).
Topics: Oral examination, complementary tests, white lesions, ulcerative lesions, proliferative lesions, vesiculobullous diseases, pigmented lesions, tongue disorders, potentially malignant disorders, oral cancer, and intraosseous lesions.
Impact Evaluation

- *2013*: The impact of the course on the participants' self-confidence to diagnose and manage oral lesions was evaluated (Fig. 9.4).

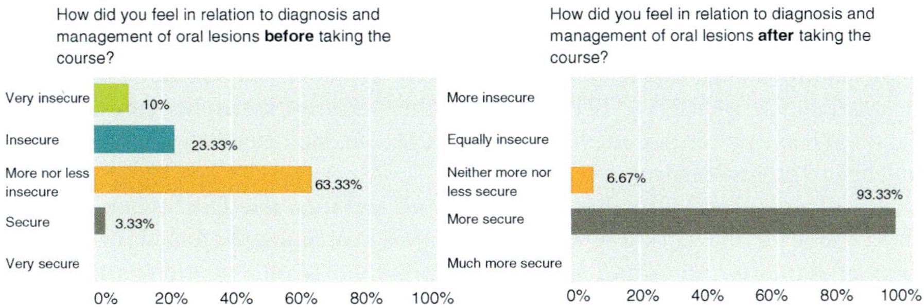

Fig. 9.4 Perception of participants ($n = 30$) of the 3rd edition of the course "Oral Medicine for Primary Health Care"

9.3.3.2 Phase 2

Format

- Flipped classroom: Participants are expected to read/study assigned materials prior to watching video classes.
- Content preparation followed the diagnostic reasoning of the specialist.
- Innovative virtual learning objects (virtual training environment): collection of images with which participants could practice their diagnostic ability (for ulcerative and white lesions only).
- Course available in an institutional e-learning platform (Moodle UFRGS).

Duration: 30 h over 12 weeks.
Target audience: 1st- and 5th-year (freshmen and senior) undergraduate students of the School of Dentistry at the Federal University of Rio Grande do Sul.
Editions: One (2016).
Topics: Oral examination, complementary tests, white lesions, ulcerative lesions, erosive lesions, proliferative lesions, vesiculobullous diseases, pigmented lesions, potentially malignant disorders, and oral cancer.
Impact evaluation: Pretest/posttest evaluation based on clinical photos of oral lesions to assess the diagnostic skills of participants. Participants had to classify the lesions as benign, potentially malignant, or malignant and formulate a clinical impression. The course resulted in a 16% increase in the ability to correctly classify the lesions and about 27% increase in right responses for clinical impression.

9.4 Telediagnosis (2015–2017)

Telediagnosis in oral medicine has been discussed for over a decade worldwide. The first study on that topic was published by Leão and Potter [15]. These authors compared digital photographs of oral lesions with their detailed description. Based on dentists' evaluation, it was possible to demonstrate that digital photographs were reliable for evaluation. Later, the accuracy of telediagnosis by means of clinical photographs was assessed. Based on clinical photos sent by e-mail, Torres-Pereira et al. [16] found relatively low agreement between two specialists. However, the authors still claimed that telediagnosis could be effective and beneficial. Recently, Petruzzi and de Benedittis [17] reported on the use of the smartphone-based application WhatsApp for oral medicine case discussion and consultation with patients and health professionals.

After some years providing teleconsulting services, the TSRS team realized that changes to the workflow were necessary. A protocol was created for submission of requests, according to which a minimum of information is required. Additionally, submission of smartphone photos became mandatory. The intention was to allow more specific and accurate responses. This step was challenging, because the protocol had to be strict but could not become discouraging or

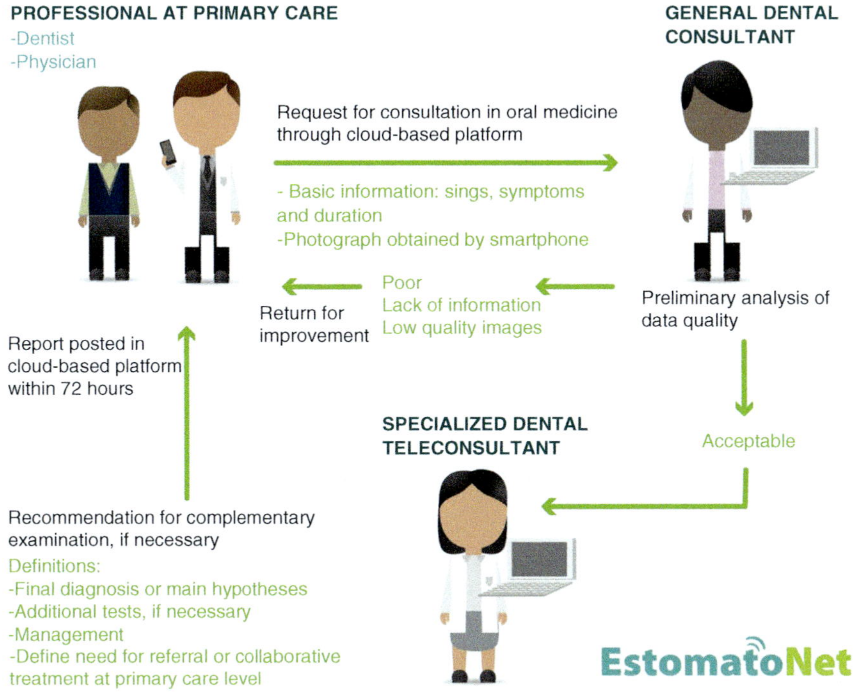

Fig. 9.5 A summary of the EstomatoNet (oral medicine net) service workflow

excessively time-consuming, which could lead to low usage by the health professionals.

Definition

– Teleconsulting to support decision-making in diagnosis and management of oral lesions, preventing unnecessary referrals to specialists.

Purpose

– To increase the number of cases treated in primary health-care settings.
– To qualify referrals, improving the information provided with the referral and defining the level of priority of each case.

Workflow (Fig. 9.5): Requester fills a form with basic information about the case (age, gender, chief complaint, removable prosthesis use, systemic disorders, use of drugs, description of the lesion, signs and symptoms, duration of lesion). Photographs made with a smartphone must be added. In order to facilitate this task, basic orientation on how to obtain proper smartphone photos is offered (Fig. 9.6). The consultant returns a report including (a) one or more diagnostic hypothesis,

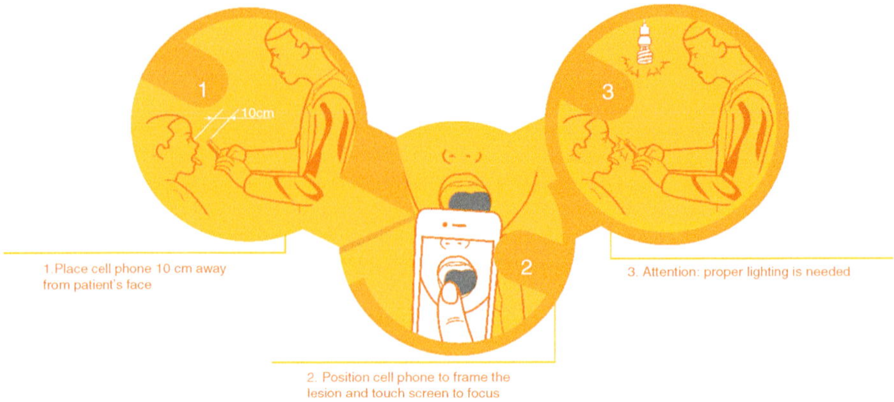

Fig. 9.6 Basic orientation on distance, position, and lighting conditions for recording clinical photos with a smartphone

(b) recommendation in relation to management/treatment of the lesion, and (c) need to refer the patient to specialist care or recommendation for treatment in PHC facilities.

Target audience: Primary care physicians and dentists.
Preliminary results (based on the first 100 requests)

- Identification of high number of cases treatable at the PHC level.
- Remarkable reduction on intention to refer the patient for face-to-face consultation with a specialist (about 38%).
- High level of user satisfaction (96%).

Pros

- Reduction of referral queue/backlog.
- Improvement in the quality of the primary care provided to patients with oral lesions.
- Improvement in the information submitted with referrals for face-to-face specialist consultation.

Cons

- The perceptions of requesters regarding the problem and the information they choose to provide may still influence the diagnostic reasoning of teleconsultants. Thus, untrained or unknowledgeable requesters may compromise the process.

9.5 RegulaSUS: An Initiative Focused on the Health-Care Work Process/Referral System (2015–2017)

Considering that the delay in diagnosis is related to poor prognosis for oral cancer, an intervention focusing on the referral system for specialized consultations was assumed to be important. In this sense, it should be emphasized that specialists in oral medicine are available in only a few cities within the public health-care system. Before the partnership with TSRS, the state referral system had no criteria to prioritize cases based on urgency.

Definition: RegulaSUS, a service created by TSRS, aims to sort the referral queue and reduce the time to specialist consultation taking into account the priority level of cases.
Format: Analysis of referrals and definition of level of priority by a dentist, according to the following classification: (P0) very high priority, corresponding to cases with diagnosis confirmed by biopsy and histopathological examination or cases suspicious for malignancy, (P1) potentially malignant lesion, and (P2) other lesions, when not treatable in PHC. The minimum set of information to be submitted for analysis was also defined:

1. Description of lesion (duration, elementary lesion, color, size, surface, consistency).
2. Related signs and symptoms.
3. If white patch: Removable by scraping (yes/not)?
4. Previous treatment: If performed, which? Provide result.
5. Biopsy: If performed, provide result.
6. Imaginologic exams: If performed, provide results.
7. EstomatoNet: If contacted, provide report.

Results

- Elimination of almost 400 requests from referral queues.
- Reduction in time to face-to-face specialist consultation from 162 to 50 days (69.14%).

Pros

- Potential impact on early diagnosis and possibly on mortality rate from oral cancer.

Cons

- Dependence on engagement of PHC professional for screening and referring patients accordingly.

9.6 Challenges and Perspectives

Early diagnosis of oral cancer and the high mortality rate associated with this cancer are complex issues. Changing this scenario depends on actions that involve education/raising awareness of the population, further training of future professionals, continuing education of professionals in the health-care network, and improvement of work processes.

Using the Internet to increase the knowledge and awareness of the population regarding their general health seems like a promising strategy. However, some barriers must be considered. The access of older people and those with lower socioeconomic status to these resources is limited. This would complicate, at least in part, the diffusion of information [18, 19]. In addition, when they search the Internet for answers to specific questions, patients do not always access websites that provide precise and reliable information [20].

Regarding oral cancer, van der Waal [4] considers that prevention is the only measure to reduce mortality rates; the most important prevention measures include reduced exposure to risk factors (tobacco use, routine alcohol consumption, and unprotected exposure to ultraviolet radiation). However, studies show that a variable and relatively low proportion of dentists routinely recommend reduced exposure to these factors [21–25]. In part, this finding may be explained by the fact that professionals perceive themselves as having limited skills to detect oral lesions [21–26]. The need to implement training to meet this demand is obvious, a gap that may be resolved by distance learning.

Despite the self-perception of health-care professionals (dentists and physicians) as unprepared or not up to date in relation to oral cancer, they do not routinely seek continuing education programs [27, 28]. Initiatives aiming at encouraging this group of unmotivated professionals to participate in education activities should be considered in order to increase the impact of other measures. The same applies to the search for interventions that produce change in the way dentistry is practiced, since 34% of dentists become skilled to detect oral lesions after they take training courses [21].

Conversely, theoretical knowledge about cancer does not seem to be directly associated with the capacity to make early diagnoses [29]. Most professionals perceive themselves as not sufficiently trained to perform an examination of the mucosa to detect oral cancer [9, 30–32]. In addition, over half the dentists do not feel safe to perform a biopsy, decreasing the possibility of diagnosis by general dental practitioners [12, 33]. In this light, it seems that training programs should provide opportunities for practical training, including in patient examination, active search of lesions, and exposure to the diagnostic challenge. This is crucial to enhance the diagnostic skill of oral health professionals.

Concerning telediagnosis, our initial experience has shown that this tool can effectively contribute to improve oral medicine care in the public health network. Until now, EstomatoNet has been accessed by professionals from 57 out of 497 municipalities in the state of Rio Grande do Sul, with increasing but still low usage. The next step will be the creation of an app to reach additional professionals and municipalities.

TSRS support of the referral system (RegulaSUS), another soft spot in health care, has shown striking results. In the near future, we will be able to evaluate the impact of this service on oral cancer prognosis and mortality rate.

Conclusion

In conclusion, some important, although preliminary, advances have been achieved in oral cancer management using information technology in the state of Rio Grande do Sul. The implementation of initiatives focused on bridging the gap in other regions and countries may produce substantial improvement in oral health issues worldwide.

References

1. Petersen PE. Oral cancer prevention and control–the approach of the World Health Organization. Oral Oncol. 2009;45(4-5):454–60.
2. Warnakulasuriya S. Global epidemiology of oral and oropharyngeal cancer. Oral Oncol. 2009;45(4-5):309–16.
3. Shield KD, et al. The global incidence of lip, oral cavity, and pharyngeal cancers by subsite in 2012. CA Cancer J Clin. 2016;67(1):51–64.
4. van der Waal I. Are we able to reduce the mortality and morbidity of oral cancer; some considerations. Med Oral Patol Oral Cir Bucal. 2013;18(1):e33–7.
5. Rogers SN, et al. Survival following primary surgery for oral cancer. Oral Oncol. 2009;45(3):201–11.
6. Guneri P, Epstein JB. Late stage diagnosis of oral cancer: components and possible solutions. Oral Oncol. 2014;50(12):1131–6.
7. McPherson LM, et al. The role of primary healthcare professionals in oral cancer prevention and detection. Br Dent J. 2003;195(5):277–81.
8. Scully C, et al. Sources and patterns of referrals of oral cancer: role of general practitioners. Br Med J. 1986;293(6547):599–601.
9. Ergun S, et al. Dentists' knowledge and opinions about oral mucosal lesions. Int J Oral Maxillofac Surg. 2009;38(12):1283–8.
10. Diamanti N, et al. Attitudes to biopsy procedures in general dental practice. Br Dent J. 2002;192(10):588–92.
11. McCann PJ, et al. Training in oral disease, diagnosis and treatment for medical students and doctors in the United Kingdom. Br J Oral Maxillofac Surg. 2005;43(1):61–4.
12. Wan A, Savage NW. Biopsy and diagnostic histopathology in dental practice in Brisbane: usage patterns and perceptions of usefulness. Aust Dent J. 2010;55(2):162–9.
13. Haberland CM, Allen CM, Beck FM. Referral patterns, lesion prevalence, and patient care parameters in a clinical oral pathology practice. Oral Surg Oral Med Oral Pathol Oral Radiol Endod. 1999;87(5):583–8.
14. Roxo-Gonçalves M, et al. Teledentistry: a tool to promote continuing education actions on oral medicine for primary healthcare professionals. Telemed J E Health. 2016;23(4):327–33.
15. Leão JC, Potter SR. Telediagnosis of oral disease. Braz Dent J. 1999;10(1):47–53.
16. Torres-Pereira CM, et al. Teledentistry: distant diagnosis of oral disease using e-mails. Telemed J E-Health. 2013;19(2):117–21.
17. Petruzzi M, de Benedittis M. WhatsApp: a telemedicine platform for facilitating remote oral medicine consultation and improving clinical examinations. Oral Surg Oral Med Oral Pathol Oral Radiol. 2016;121(3):248–54.
18. Paul CL, et al. Improving access to information and support for patients with less common cancers: hematologic cancer patients' views about Web-based approaches. J Med Internet Res. 2011;13(4):e112.

19. Wilson C, et al. Internet access for delivery of health information to South Australians older than 50. Aust N Z J Public Health. 2008;32(2):174–6.
20. McMullan M. Patients using the Internet to obtain health information: how this affects the patient-health professional relationship. Patient Educ Couns. 2006;63(1-2):24–8.
21. Gajendra S, Cruz GD, Kumar JV. Oral cancer prevention and early detection: knowledge, practices, and opinions of oral health care providers in New York State. J Cancer Educ. 2006;21(3):157–62.
22. Kujan O, et al. Opinions and attitudes of the UK's GDPs and specialists in oral surgery, oral medicine and surgical dentistry on oral cancer screening. Oral Dis. 2006;12(2):194–9.
23. Seoane-Leston J, et al. Knowledge of oral cancer and preventive attitudes of Spanish dentists. Primary effects of a pilot educational intervention. Med Oral Patol Oral Cir Bucal. 2010;15(3):e422–6.
24. Seoane J, et al. Oral cancer: experiences and diagnostic abilities elicited by dentists in North-Western Spain. Oral Dis. 2006;12(5):487–92.
25. Warnakulasuriya KA, Nanayakkara BG. Reproducibility of an oral cancer and precancer detection program using a primary health care model in Sri Lanka. Cancer Detect Prev. 1991;15(5):331–4.
26. Alonge OK, Narendran S. Opinions about oral cancer prevention and early detection among dentists practising along the Texas-Mexico border. Oral Dis. 2003;9(1):41–5.
27. Hassona Y, et al. Oral cancer early detection--a pressing need for continuing education in Jordan. Asian Pac J Cancer Prev. 2015;16(17):7727–30.
28. Hassona Y, et al. Oral cancer knowledge and diagnostic ability among dental students. J Cancer Educ. 2015;32(3):566–70.
29. Hassona Y, et al. Factors influencing early detection of oral cancer by primary health-care professionals. J Cancer Educ. 2016;31(2):285–91.
30. Hertrampf K, et al. Early detection of oral cancer: dentists' opinions and practices before and after educational interventions in Northern-Germany. J Craniomaxillofac Surg. 2013;41(8):e201–7.
31. Razavi SM, et al. Dentists' knowledge, attitude, and practice regarding oral cancer in Iran. J Cancer Educ. 2013;28(2):335–41.
32. Shimpi N, et al. Knowledgeability, attitude and behavior of primary care providers towards oral cancer: a pilot study. J Cancer Educ. 2016. https://doi.org/10.1007/s13187-016-1084-4.
33. Lopez Jornet P, et al. Attitude towards oral biopsy among general dentists in Murcia. Med Oral Patol Oral Cir Bucal. 2007;12(2):E116–21.

Part III

A Global View on Teledentistry

Teledentistry in the United States

10

Susan J. Daniel and Lindsie Farrow

Abstract

This chapter provides an overview of the history, development, and influences on the adoption of teledentistry in the United States. The United States does not have a national healthcare system. Each state has oversight for healthcare through professional and health regulatory agencies. Adoption of teledentistry by states is increasing due to governmental influences to improve access to care. Reimbursement for services performed with teledentistry is more common for children through Medicare and less so for adults; however, new treatment codes for teledentistry examinations are available. Continued expansion of teledentistry is imminent with advances in technology, and in intraprofessional and interprofessional collaborations.

Keywords

History • Adoption • Collaborative care

10.1 Introduction

A brief review of the development of dentistry in the United States is required to understand the development of teledentistry. Baltimore College of Dental Surgery, the first School of Dentistry, opened in 1840, and the American Dental Association (ADA) was established in 1859. The first school of dental hygiene was established in Bridgeport, Connecticut, in 1913, and 10 years later (1923), the American Dental Hygienists' Association (ADHA) was established. The ADA and the

S.J. Daniel (✉)
School of Dental Hygiene, Old Dominion University, Norfolk, VA, USA
e-mail: sjdaniel@odu.edu

L. Farrow
Southern Dominion Health System, Inc., Victoria, VA, USA

N. Giraudeau (ed.), *e-Health Care in Dentistry and Oral Medicine*,
https://doi.org/10.1007/978-3-319-69450-4_10

ADHA are the national professional organizations of dentistry and dental hygiene, respectively. The Commission on Dental and Allied Dental Accreditation (CODA) prescribes the standards for dental, dental hygiene, dental therapy, dental assisting, and dental laboratory educational programs as well as dental specialty programs.

Each state has legal jurisdiction over licensing and practice of dental care within their jurisdiction. In some states there are separate regulatory boards for dentistry and dental hygiene; however, the majority of regulatory oversight for all oral care providers resides within a state's dental board. Boards of Dentistry are comprised primarily of dental providers. Recently, the US Federal Trade Commission has been involved in challenging the scope of dental boards and the restrictions on the delivery of oral care by other providers such as licensed dental hygienists and dental therapists.

10.2 Development of Teledentistry

The "Total Dental Access Project" implemented by the Army in 1994 is the first reported use of teledentistry in the United States. The project was developed to reduce cost for dental services and to increase access in rural and remote locations [1]. Following the Army's use of teledentistry, the University of Southern California's Mobile Dental Clinic partnered with the Children's Hospital Los Angeles in a teledentistry project to serve children in remote areas [2].

Shortly thereafter, the University of Minnesota recognized the need to use teledentistry for consultations and referrals with underserved families and partnered with Hibbing Community College in this effort. Another model emerged for the use of teledentistry when the Alaskan Native Tribal Health Consortium developed the Dental Health Aid Therapist (DHAT) in collaboration with the University of Washington in 2007. Dental therapists perform preventive and restorative services and consult with dental and other healthcare providers through teledentistry [3].

A pivotal program emerged in California known as the "Virtual Dental Home," and in 2015, the California general assembly passed a bill to allow for the training of dental hygienists to be part of a teledentistry team in rural and underserved populations [4]. This bill permits a dental hygienist to perform preventive and restorative procedures in community settings while consulting remotely with dentists regarding treatment.

Arizona also approved licensed dental hygienists provision of oral care services to the underserved without general or direct supervision from a dentist. The Northern Arizona University (NAU) Dental Hygiene Department created and successfully demonstrated a teledentistry-assisted dental hygiene model. This model digitally connects all physically separated members of a teledentistry team, meeting the federal government's call for an alternative dental healthcare workforce [5].

The Affordable Care Act requirements to address the unmet healthcare needs of many have been instrumental in changing access to oral care, increasing the scope of practice of licensed providers, development of dental therapists, and expanding the use of teledentistry and telehealth technologies. Each state was contacted to obtain current information on the status of teledentistry. Most responded or content was obtained through an Internet search. Table 10.1 provides a list of all states with the status of teledentistry at the time of this publication.

Reimbursement for telehealth services has been a barrier for adoption, but that is changing. Data obtained by the Center for Connected Health Policy (CCHP) publishes trends on telehealth law and reimbursement for medical providers specifically related to Medicaid reimbursement. The Center recently reported that 46 states have a form of reimbursement for telehealth applications in their public programs [6]. Reimbursement for teledentistry is more likely to come through Medicaid than private insurers; however, codes applicable to teledentistry have been added to the CDT 2016 Dental Procedure Codes [7]. States have been much slower in approving teledentistry and measures for reimbursement.

Table 10.1 Teledentistry status by state

State	Status	State	Status
Alabama	Yes	Nebraska	Yes by University of Nebraska
Alaska	Yes	Nevada	Yes
Arizona	Yes	New Hampshire	No
Arkansas	No	New Jersey	No
California	Yes	New Mexico	Yes
Colorado	Yes	New York	Yes
Connecticut	Yes	North Carolina	No
Delaware	Yes	North Dakota	No
District of Columbia	No	Ohio	No
Florida	Yes	Oklahoma	Yes
Georgia	Yes	Oregon	Yes
Hawaii	Yes	Pennsylvania	No
Idaho	No	Rhode Island	No
Illinois	No	South Carolina	No
Indiana	Bill submitted	South Dakota	Yes
Iowa	No	Texas	Yes
Kansas	No	Utah	No
Kentucky	Yes	Vermont	No
Louisiana	No	Virginia	Pilot program
Maine	No	Washington	Yes by Native American Tribe
Massachusetts	No	West Virginia	No
Minnesota	Yes	Wisconsin	No
Mississippi	Yes	Wyoming	No
Missouri	Bill waiting for Governor's signature		
Montana	No		

10.3 Influences on Adoption

The recognition of the number of citizens without oral care due to access issues, no dental insurance and health literacy concerns, coupled with the rise in dental caries among young children and subsets of the population such as those in long-term care facilities, has illuminated the need for greater access and the use of teledentistry. Teledentistry and an expanded workforce could address the 46 million Americans living in designated dental shortage areas [8].

Reports from the Institute of Medicine and Health and Human Services brought more visibility to the need for access and reduction of practice restrictions on licensed allied dental personnel to meet the oral health needs of the population [9, 10]. Further epidemiological data from the National Health and Nutrition Examination Survey (NHANES) illuminated the continued high caries rate among young children (23% aged 2–5 with caries) and the populations with greatest oral disease and unmet needs (Hispanic and non-Hispanic Blacks aged 2–8) [11].

Added to the data from national studies and reports are the US governmental influencers such as the Patient Protection and Affordable Care Act 2010 (ACA) and the meaningful use incentive for adoption of electronic health records [12]. Requirements outlined in the ACA produced change in the delivery of oral care as shown by (1) a reduction in practice restrictions for licensed allied dental professionals, (2) direct access to patients, and (3) remote consultation or supervision with a dentist through teledentistry technology.

Another measure to increase use of teledentistry is the "meaningful use" incentive. The American Recovery and Reinvestment Act (ARRA) was enacted on February 17, 2009 [13]. Title XIII of ARRA is the "Health Information Technology for Economic and Clinical Health Act" which seeks to improve the delivery of healthcare in the United States by incentivizing the implementation and meaningful use of electronic health records (EHRs).

The Health and Human Services Office of Health Reform and the Center for Medicare and Medicaid Services issued the requirement that all medical and dental offices convert to an electronic health record system by 2016, thus allowing for participation in the incentive program. Meaningful use and the stages are implemented to carry out core requirements to insure proper data is being recorded in electronic medical and dental records.

Perhaps the most influential measure on adoption of teledentistry to date could be the November 2015 policy passed by the American Dental Association's House of Delegates stating that teledentistry is a method for delivering a service [14]. The policy includes what patients can expect when receiving teledentistry services, licensure of providers, and payment and types of teledentistry technologies. The policy also addressed mobile healthcare and communications including apps to assist and monitor a patient's oral care.

As a result of the ADA policy on teledentistry, governmental influences, and epidemiological data illuminating the unmet oral care needs of the population, educational institutions must prepare oral care providers to work with telehealth technologies. The American Dental Association's Commission on Dental Accreditation standards require educational programs to prepare students to be clinically competent in functions identified in the practice act of each respective state. Curricular modifications are necessary in dental and allied dental educational programs with increased adoption of teledentistry measures in the delivery of oral care.

An additional element that could influence teledentistry is to become more integrated into the health system with medical care. Telemedicine or telehealth in the United States has been adopted in some form by 46 states with an active American Telemedicine Association. A similar association could be formed to meet the unique needs of oral care in this emerging telehealth world. Lessons learned from the telemedicine association could be adopted.

10.4 Future

Technology has and will continue to change the way oral care needs are met. Patients will become more active in their health with the use of mobile phones, photography, and access to their health records; and thereby, professionals have the ability to improve health literacy. Dental care delivery must change to meet the needs of the populace. Regulations in healthcare are necessary for the protection of those we serve; however, some regulations can prohibit the acquisition and delivery of needed, timely care by competent licensed professionals using the technologies available for consultation with multiple healthcare professionals.

Conclusion

Change is difficult, but change is inevitable, and without it, professions, professionals, and society become stagnant and individuals languish without needed care increasing financial burdens to individuals, third-party payers, and governments. The integration of oral care into general healthcare is underway in the United States through interprofessional educational initiatives and collaborative practice models that employ telehealth measures. These models are dynamic and engage patients with a collaborative healthcare team to meet the diverse needs of the expanding population.

References

1. Rocca MA, Kudryk VL, Pajak JC, Morris Tommy. The evolution of teledentistry system within the Department of Defense. National Institues of Health, Bethesda, MD; 1999. p. 921–23. http://www.ncbi.nlm.nih.gov/pmc/articles/PMC2232632/pdf/procamiasymp00004-0958.pdf. 27 June 2016.
2. Chang S, Plotkin D, Mulligan R, et al. Teledentistry in rural California: a USC initiative. Calif Dent Assoc J. 2003;31(8):601–8. http://www.ncbi.nlm.nih.gov/pubmed/13677402. Accessed 28 June 2016.

3. Willard ME. AlaskaTribal Health System Oral Health. In: Consortium ANTH, editor. Alaska; 2013. http://dhss.alaska.gov/ahcc/Documents/meetings/201303/AlaskaTribalHealth-OralHealth-Williard.pdf. Accessed 28 June 2016.
4. Healthline Medi-Cal to cover teledentistry services beginning in 2015. California; 2014. http://californiahealthline.org/morning-breakout/medical-to-cover-teledentistry-services-beginning-in-2015/. Accessed 28 June 2016.
5. Summerfeldt FF. Teledentistry-assisted, affiliated practice for dental hygienists: an innovative oral health workforce model. J Dent Educ. 2011;75(6):733–42. http://www.ncbi.nlm.nih.gov/pubmed/21642518. Accessed 28 June 2016.
6. Center for Connected Health Policy: The National Telehealth Policy Resource Center. State Telehealth Laws and Reimbursement Policies: a comprehensive scan of the 50 States and District of Columbia; 2015. http://cchpca.org/sites/default/files/resources/State Laws and Reimbursement Policies Report Feb 2015.pdf. Accessed 28 June 16.
7. America Dental Association. CDT 2016 dental procedure codes. Chicago: American Dental Association; 2016. http://www.ada.org/en/publications/ada-catalog/cdt-products. Accessed 28 June 16.
8. Designated shortage areas: health professional shortage areas & medically underserved areas/populations. U.S. Department of Health and Human Services, Health Resource Services Administration; 2013. http://datawarehouse.hrsa.gov/. Accessed 27 June 2016.
9. Institute of Medicine. Improving Access to Oral Health Care for Vulnerable and Underserved Populations. The National Academies of Sciences, Engineering and Medicine. Washington DC; 2011. http://nationalacademies.org/hmd/reports/2011/improving-access-to-oral-health-care-for-vulnerable-and-underserved-populations.aspx. Accessed 27 June 2016.
10. United States Department of Health and Human Services (DHHS). National call to action to promote oral health. Rockville, MD: National Institute of Dental and Craniofacial Research; 2003, Spring. http://www.nidcr.nih.gov/DataStatistics/SurgeonGeneral/NationalCalltoAction. Accessed 27 June 2016.
11. Dye BA, Tan S, Smith V. Trends in Oral Health Status: United States, 1988–1994 and 1999–2004. National Center for Health Statistics. Health and Human Services. Centers for Disease Control, Washington, D.C.; April 2007. https://www.cdc.gov/nchs/data/series/sr_11/sr11_248.pdf. Accessed 27 June 16.
12. United States Congress. Patient Protection and Affordable Care Act. 42 U.S.C. § 18001 et seq. (2010). United States 2010. https://www.gpo.gov/fdsys/pkg/PLAW-111publ148/pdf/PLAW-111publ148.pdf. Accessed 27 June 2016.
13. United States Congress. American Recovery and Reinvestment Act of 2009. First Session, January 6, 2009. Washington, D.C. Page. H.R.1–112–H.R.1–165. https://www.gpo.gov/fdsys/pkg/BILLS-111hr1enr/pdf/BILLS-111hr1enr.pdf. Accessed 27 June 2016.
14. American Dental Association. House of delegates passes guidelines on teledentistry. Chicago: ADA; 2015. http://www.ada.org/en/publications/ada-news/2015-archive/december/house-passes-guidelines-on-teledentistry. Accessed 28 June 16.

Teledentistry in Brazil: Tools to Improve the Quality of Oral Health in the Primary Care Setting

11

Otávio Pereira D'Avila, Cynthia Goulart Molina-Bastos, Rafael Gustavo dal Moro, Erno Harzheim, Marcelo Rodrigues Gonçalves, Roberto Nunes Umpierre, Carlos André Aita Shmitz, and Vinicius Coelho Carrard

Abstract

The use of telehealth tools in Brazil has been increasing in recent years. Specifically in dentistry, use has been more associated with e-learning actions. More recently there has been investment in teleconsulting actions and support for clinical decision making from web based systems and app development. Although there is still a long way to go brazilian e-health already presents good reports of it use in three broad areas: teleconsulting, telediagnosis and e-learning.

Keywords

E-health • Telehealth and dentistry

O.P. D'Avila (✉) • C.G. Molina-Bastos • R.G. dal Moro
TelessaúdeRS/UFRGS, Porto Alegre, Brazil
e-mail: otaviopereiradavila@gmail.com

E. Harzheim
School of Medicine, Federal University of Rio Grande do Sul, Porto Alegre, Brazil

M.R. Gonçalves • R.N. Umpierre • C.A.A. Shmitz
TelessaúdeRS/UFRGS, Porto Alegre, Brazil
School of Medicine, Federal University of Rio Grande do Sul, Porto Alegre, Brazil

V.C. Carrard
TelessaúdeRS/UFRGS, Porto Alegre, Brazil
School of Dentistry, Federal University of Rio Grande do Sul, Porto Alegre, Brazil

N. Giraudeau (ed.), *e-Health Care in Dentistry and Oral Medicine*,
https://doi.org/10.1007/978-3-319-69450-4_11

11.1 Introduction

In the last 15 years, Brazil has invested in the development of oral health services for Primary Health Care (PHC). In 2002 there were 4261 oral health teams linked to PHC, in 2017 there were 24,053 [1–4]. This investment reflected directly in the expansion of access to oral health services that reached the mark of more than 74 million people covered by these services. However, there are still some challenges to be solved in order to increase the resolution of these services. Lack of structure as adequate materials, access to complementary exams as well as deficiencies in academic training can be pointed out as some of the reasons [3, 4].

Few initiatives at the national level have been developed to address this scenario. In 2007, following the launch of the National Telehealth Program, some initiatives support the qualification and increase of the resolution of oral health services through telehealth tools. The program aims to improve the quality of care, increase the scope of actions offered by teams, and increase clinical capacity, from the development of actions to support health care and e-learning for PHC teams. There are 26 health care centers in Brazil, in stages or differentiated service development. The actions offered involve teleconsultation, telediagnosis, and e-learning. Although in slow development, they are continuous actions that point to a promising future of teleodontology in Brazil.

This chapter aims to describe the tele-health services in dentistry developed in Brazil for primary health care professionals in Brazil.

11.2 Oral Health in the Primary Care Setting in Brazil: State of the Art

For many years, oral health care in Brazil was only available through private insurance or to workers contributing to the National Institute of Medical Care and Social Security INAMPS [1]. This restrictive model generated a gap between socioeconomic classes, which began to be tackled only recently with the inclusion of oral health in the model of primary health care (PHC).

In 1998, the Brazilian National Household Sample Survey (PNAD) revealed that an estimated 29.6 million people (18.7% of the Brazilian population) had never been examined by a dentist. The PNAD also detected an important effect of household income on the access to [oral] health services: the percentage who had never been to a dentist was nine times higher in households earning up to one minimum salary as compared to those earning more than 20 minimum salaries.

In 2003, oral health became part of the national PHC strategy with the launch of the National Oral Health Policy—Smiling Brazil [2]. Initially, the policy expanded oral health services at the primary care level, with the aim of increasing access. It also established guidelines that shifted the focus of oral health services toward PHC initiatives and attributes [3]. Over than 10 years later, there is concrete evidence of the significant expansion in oral health coverage. As of April 2003, around 4500 PHC teams included a dentist; currently, more than 25,700 teams have a dentist member [4].

Despite the inclusion of oral health as part of the PHC system in Brazil, disparities in access are still present [5], and the resolvability of a wide range of primary care procedures is still limited [6, 7]. Also, fragmented care coordination is directly related to the still incipient character of the oral health-care network in Brazil. Even though the National Oral Health Policy mandates the creation of referral flows between levels of care [8], the number of referral facilities is insufficient to meet the demand generated by the Policy [9].

Thus, it is essential to strengthen the delivery of primary oral health care in Brazil. In this context, telehealth tools may be key to increase resolvability and improve the coordination of care.

11.3 Telehealth Brazil Networks

Brazil began to invest in public telehealth policies in 2007 with the creation of nine telehealth groups based in federal universities. Since then, several phases of the Telehealth Brazil Networks Program have been implemented, including the creation of interstate and inter-municipal telehealth groups. As of 2015, 22 states were involved, and 38 telehealth groups were active in the country [10].

Despite the overall focus on PHC support, many telehealth groups have specialized in specific tools or initiatives. In the states of Santa Catarina and Rio de Janeiro, emphasis was placed on telediagnosis and tele-radiology. One group in the state of Minas Gerais dedicated itself to tele-education tools, while a second group developed expertise in telediagnosis and electrocardiology (pioneer service in Brazil). In the state of São Paulo, a group focused on tele-education and the production of complex learning objects (e.g., Virtual Human Project). In the state of Amazonas, in addition to the attention to specific demands relating to indigenous peoples, a group addressed the geographic characteristics of the region and became experienced in conducting actions with special data transmission structures, given the limited availability of health-care professionals at points of care [11].

The initiatives developed in oral medicine have included teleconsulting, telediagnosis, and tele-education actions.

11.4 Teleconsulting

Teleconsulting [in oral medicine] is mainly used to provide support for care, promoting discussions among peers for resolution of clinical questions. Teleconsultations must be based on the best available evidence and adapted for the context of the requester. Expected outcomes of teleconsulting are increase in the capacity of requesters to resolve health issues at the primary care level, improvement in the quality of the information that accompanies referrals for specialist care, and prevention of unnecessary referrals. In fact, one out of two teleconsultations requested by medical professionals ends with a decision not to refer the patient for specialist care [12–14]. Teleconsulting also works as a tool for continuing education or continuing professional development—this is because the discussion of cases may produce changes in clinical behaviors.

According to the legal framework established by the Brazilian Ministry of Health, teleconsulting is defined as a “recorded exchange among health-care workers, professionals, and managers, using bidirectional telecommunication tools, with the aim of resolving doubts about clinical procedures, health actions, and questions relating to the work process, and divided into two types: (a) synchronous, real-time teleconsulting, usually through chats, web, or videoconference, or (b) asynchronous, provided through off-line messaging [15]".

One of the advantages of asynchronous (text) teleconsulting is the opportunity to receive a well-documented but condensed response (a maximum of one page is recommended), with references that can be further explored by the requester if desired. Conversely, real-time teleconsulting allows direct contact among more than one requester and one or more teleconsultants. These encounters must be recorded (audio or transcription) for future examination. The Ministry of Health establishes a maximum of 72 h for the elaboration of written responses and for the scheduling of real-time teleconsulting sessions (with a maximum of 72 h after live sessions for the release of the recorded exchange) [13, 15].

It is important to have professionals from the same field and level of care as the requester acts as teleconsultants. For PHC, the intervention of a specialist teleconsultant is required in only 10–20% of cases. To prevent responses based on evidence filtered for populations that are not relevant for the context of the requester (and, therefore, to prevent iatrogenic situations, which may have strong epidemiologic impact), many telehealth groups chose to introduce the role of regulator. This professional has the task of evaluating the requests to select the best teleconsultant for each case, sometimes also contributing with guidance and suggestions for the response. In addition to regulation, some groups have chosen to audit responses, which is generally done on a random sample or triggered by specific events, such as low user satisfaction levels or deviant parameters in terms of response size or time to respond. Audits are performed as a tool for peer monitoring and continuing service qualification, identifying opportunities for improvement [13, 16, 17].

At the early times of teleconsulting in Brazil, e-mail servers and text editors were used for the exchanges between requesters and teleconsultants. The first telehealth platforms (using dedicated software, with security and encryption features) became functional around 2005. In 2012, a National Telehealth Platform was launched, developed by the Rio Grande do Sul Telehealth Group (TelessaúdeRS) in partnership with the Ministry of Health. This universal access platform is available at no cost to all telehealth groups in Brazil. As of 2017, the national platform is used by 26 telehealth groups that provide support to about 53,000 health professionals (including dentists, physicians, nurses, physical therapists, dietitians, psychologists, etc.) and answer 3700 monthly requests with the help of 510 teleconsultants [10].

Some state platforms and most of the telehealth groups using the National Telehealth Platform provide access to all workers in PHC regardless of professional category or level or education. In most platforms, requests can be expressed as simple questions in free-text fields. Discussions can focus on clinical cases, specific health themes, management aspects, or work processes. Discussions through videoconference may require scheduling. Since 2013, TelessaúdeRS/UFRGS has provided 642 asynchronous teleconsultations in oral health for PHC, with a user satisfaction of 98% (Fig. 11.1).

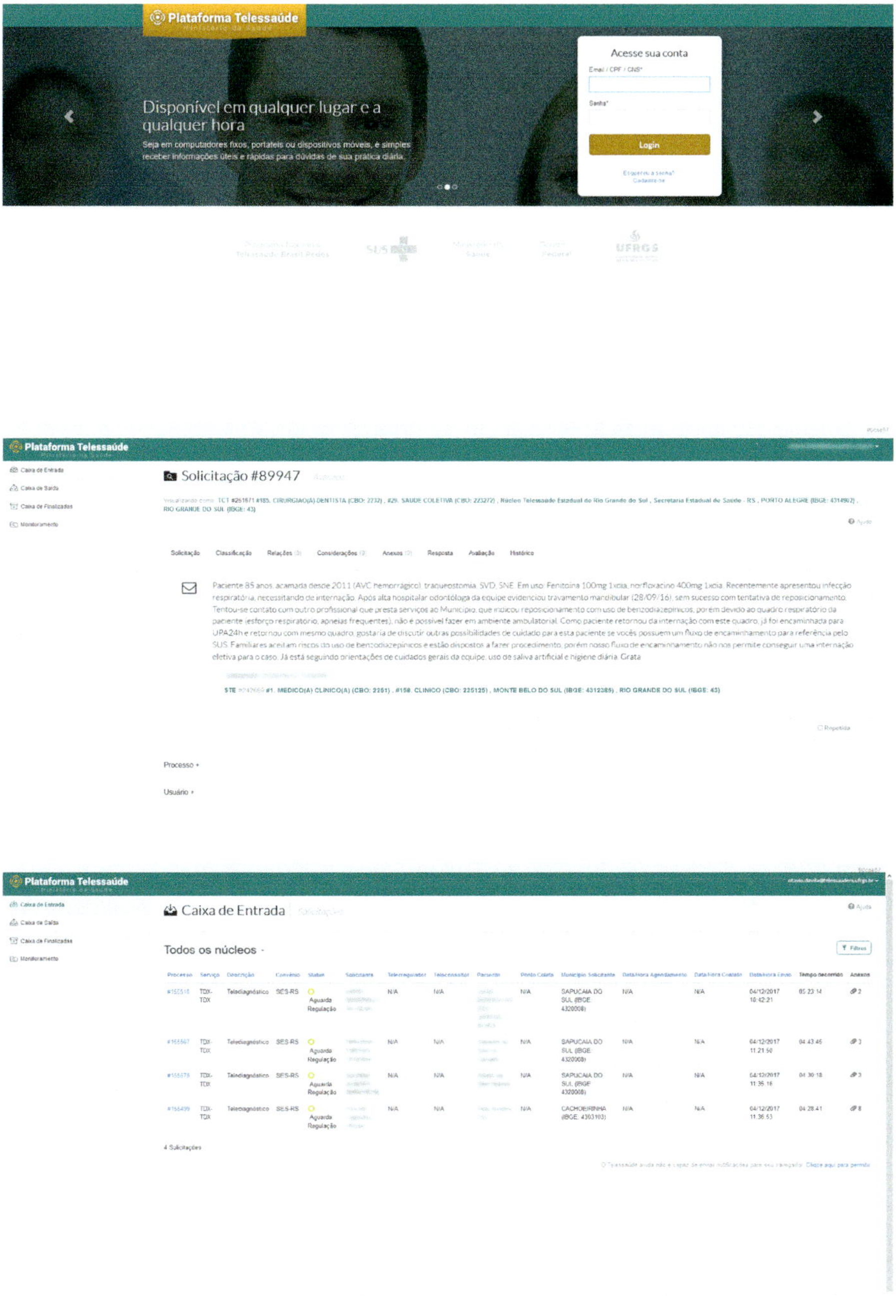

Fig. 11.1 National Telehealth Platform, version 2.0. Login, mailbox, request, and response screens. TelessaúdeRS/UFRGS, Porto Alegre, 2017

Even though the number of telehealth groups—38—seems to reflect a strength of the strategy, the installed capacity is actually idle. Perhaps as a result of the time required to formulate the questions, which has to be deducted from clinical work hours, the lack of equipment, or because of problems that are intrinsic to each requester, the number of teleconsultations is still low [18].

Also, since connectivity is limited in some regions of Brazil, the telephone has been the preferred technology for many physicians and nurses. The telephone is readily accessible even in the most remote corners of the country. To counter the impact of the low use of teleconsulting and improve accessibility for professionals from areas with limited connectivity, in 2014 the Ministry of Health launched an additional telehealth channel, a toll-free hotline available to all physicians and nurses from the entire PHC network in Brazil. By dialing 0800 644 6543, professionals can reach teleconsultants working with TelessaúdeRS/UFRGS, PHC specialists, and specialists from many other priority fields. The service is accessible during the same hours of operation of PHC units—which in Brazil usually means from 8 am to 5 pm, with the exception of special locations with specific characteristics. Calls are free from both standard lines and mobile phones. Specifically for oral medicine, the model was implemented by the telehealth group in the state of Bahia. The results of this initiative have not yet been released.

11.5 Telediagnosis

As defined in the legal framework [15], telediagnosis in Brazil is an independent health service that employs information and communication technologies to provide diagnostic support over time (not in real time) to geographically removed locations.

In Brazil, telediagnosis in oral medicine is available for oral diseases, maxillofacial surgery, pediatric dentistry, and radiology. Of these, only the data relating to oral diseases are publicly available (see chapter on oral diseases). These diagnoses are performed by TelessaúdeRS/UFRGS, which issued more than 100 reports in 2016, with a user satisfaction rate higher than 95%.

11.6 Tele-education

PHC in Brazil has gone through many changes, especially considering the significant growth in the number of teams and population coverage. This expansion has not always been matched by investments in adequate infrastructure and professional training to reach the desired resolvability potential of PHC. Thus, the need for continuing education has become increasingly evident in health care, given that the fast growth of work spaces has translated into the need of professional actions guided by knowledge and development of decision-making competencies and skills. Distance learning is a useful and strategic tool for the education of PHC workers in a country as large as Brazil [19–22].

Broadly, distance learning is a mode of instruction that employs human mediation and systematically organized didactic resources that explore different media, made available through various means of communication [14]. Technology is an important ally to shorten distances and establish a communication channel between those who produce knowledge—instructors/teleconsultants—and those who will absorb knowledge, students/requesters. Technological elements include computers, smartphones, broadband connections, and audiovisual recordings or multimedia resources for transmission of voice as well as nonverbal language. The challenge of developing education programs that contemplate discussions involving the daily routine of PHC, based on real-life problems, should guide the development of tele-education products. The development of education products is based on learning objects (LO). LOs may be defined as any modular entity, digital or non-digital, that may be used and reused for learning, education, or training. LOs are planned and built according to the objective proposed for each theme. They encompass a range of resources, from text, images, multimedia presentations, and digital film to more refined apps [13, 23].

For the purposes of the present discussion, tele-education products will be didactically divided into web lectures, courses, formative second opinion, and other modalities of case discussion employing telehealth tools.

11.7 Web Lectures

Web lectures involve communication between a speaker and an open group of participants using videoconferencing. Interaction among participants and between participants and the speaker is assumed, with exchange (usually through a chat channel) of questions and remarks. Web lectures can be used for discussion of important public health themes that need timely updates (e.g., new protocols) or cases in which there is debate regarding the best conduct to be adopted if the available evidence is not conclusive. Also, this modality is useful in public health emergencies, in which the communication of recommendations in timely manner to large numbers of professionals is advantageous (e.g., oral health for babies and children in PHC). In Brazil, ten telehealth groups have reported the performance of at least one web lecture/year for PHC dentists.

11.8 E-Learning

E-learning courses address clinical or managerial themes that pose a difficulty for PHC professionals. One way of defining the most appropriate themes for each cycle is the evaluation of [teleconsulting] requests placed by PHC workers. Usually, these consulting requests reflect situations that professionals find difficult to resolve in the PHC setting. Courses must be of short duration and focused on specific themes. Their development must be based on the best evidence available and involve LOs that use different types of media (video, text, comics, articles). LO interactivity is an essential element to attract the attention of participating professionals. Another relevant aspect is related to the format of videos: they must be short (maximum 5 min), direct, and preferably provide a practical description of the topic in the workplace. This format is more effective for learning than traditional videos using a lecturer.

Pedagogical support is a tele-education structure that aims at preventing dropout. All professionals taking a course must have their learning itinerary monitored so that any difficulties in access to virtual environments as well as learning difficulties or other limitations can be resolved with the help of pedagogical support. It should be noted that the learning itinerary should be as flexible as possible, allowing participating professionals to adapt the classes to their daily routine as they wish. Therefore, it is important to avoid a large number of synchronous (real-time) activities. For example, during a 40-h course, videoconferencing for case discussion/clarification of doubts will not be used more than twice.

Most telehealth groups, and especially those associated with a university, have a course calendar including usual and/or new courses.

In 2016, the following topics were covered in oral health:

- Oral diseases
- Pediatric dentistry
- Oral health for older adults
- Oral health in PHC

Many challenges still remain. Recent studies have shown that distance learning tools are successful in disseminating and aggregating knowledge for participating professionals, but these studies were unable to evaluate changes in professional practice or patient health outcomes over time. This suggests the need for further studies in this field and also shows that tele-education must be used as a complementary tool for other initiatives, such as teleconsulting and telediagnosis actions [18].

11.9 App Development

Information made available on smartphones to support decision-making is a useful tool for PHC professionals. In many clinical situations, information based on the best available evidence can be compiled in an app to help professionals in screening, diagnosing, and making treatment decisions for various health conditions. For that, apps must be produced using standardized development and testing processes.

TelessaúdeRS/UFRGS has developed several free apps which are made available in partnership with the Ministry of Health. The apps, which are available for Android© and iOS©, have been downloaded 400,000 times between 2015 and 2017 (Fig. 11.2).

Two apps catering to PHC dentists, for support in clinical decision-making, are currently in their final stage of development (Fig. 11.3).

11.10 Formative Second Opinion

The categorization of formative second opinion (FSO) as a subtype of teleconsulting and a tele-education product was standardized in 2014 through a specific technical note. FSOs are LOs developed from teleconsultations were provided to PHC professionals. All teleconsultations are evaluated regarding their potential as FSO. Those

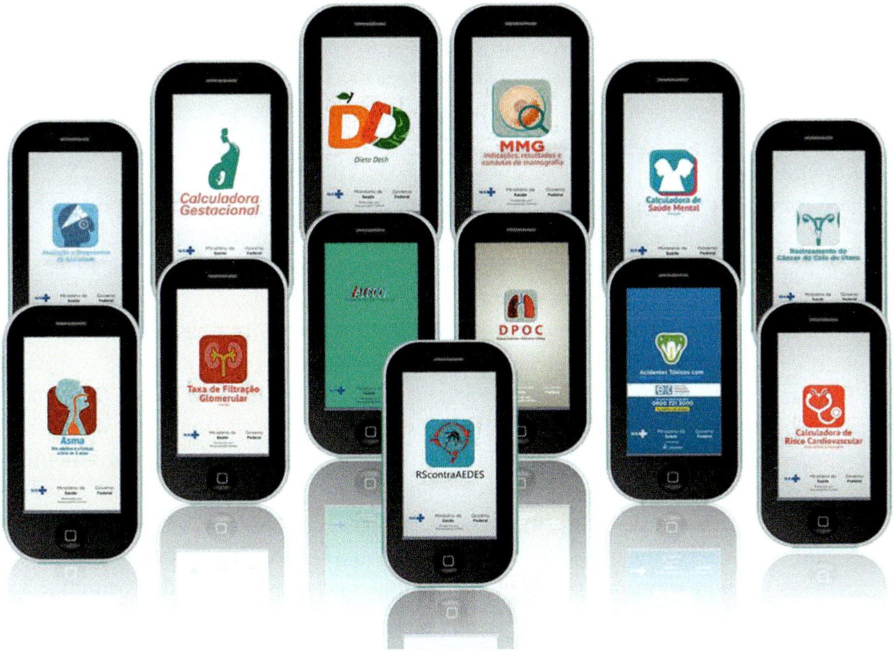

Fig. 11.2 Free apps distributed by TelessaúdeRS/UFRGS for Android© and iOS©, TelessaúdeRS/UFRGS, 2016

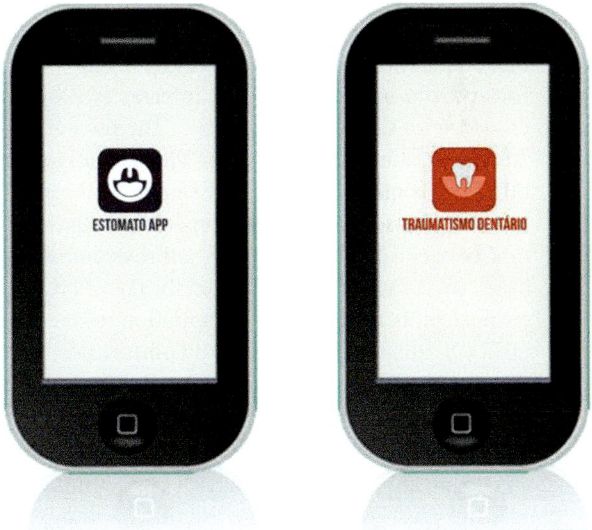

Fig. 11.3 Free [oral health] apps in final stage of development by TelessaúdeRS/UFRGS for Android© and iOS©, TelessaúdeRS/UFRGS, 2017

with greater clinical relevance for the context of PHC in Brazil are selected, structured as FSO, and forwarded for publication by the Virtual Health Library (aps.bvs.br). As of March 2017, 91 FSOs had been developed for oral PHC. In addition, 273 virtual LOs had been made available in public virtual catalogs.

Conclusion

In Brazil, investments in tele-oral medicine are insufficient to meet the needs of this area. Most telehealth groups provide asynchronous teleconsulting and distance learning in oral medicine. However, the oral health needs at the PHC and other levels of care are much greater.

Oral health-care networks encompass PHC (main point of entry into the system), specialized care in Oral Health Specialty Centers, and hospital level care. Telehealth services play an important role in strengthening oral PHC, increasing its resolvability. Emphasis should be placed on:

- Synchronous teleconsulting: The use of remote face-to-face communication tools may increase the potential of teleconsulting services in Brazil. Dentistry is often characterized by invasive procedures, and thus text or asynchronous guidance may not be sufficient. Real-time case discussions with specialists, with visualization of procedures, may translate into increased confidence for PHC dentists.
- Telediagnosis: The initial experience with telediagnosis of oral diseases indicates that the use of this technology may be essential for early diagnosis and treatment in the context of PHC, reducing the number of referrals for specialist consultations. Telediagnostic radiology may also be of interest for oral medicine.
- Tele-regulation: Patient referral for specialized and hospital services must be regulated by a specialist. Many referrals are related to oral health conditions that should be addressed at the PHC level. Using clinical protocols developed for specific specialties, each referral is reevaluated and, if necessary, discussed with the referring dentist. The resolution of the case at the PHC level is supported by teleconsulting. This initiative is already in place in Brazil for other fields of medicine. The example of TelessaúdeRS/UFRGS, which regulates referrals for 13 medical specialties, having regulated over 68,000 referrals between November 2013 and December 2016, shows that out of three cases discussed, two can be resolved in PHC. User satisfaction, rated by the requesters, is at 98%. In the regulation initiatives supported by TelessaúdeRS/UFRGS, 98% of clinicians feel comfortable being approached by teleconsultants, and 97% state that the way they practice medicine changed after they came in contact with telehealth tools.

Major hurdles to increasing the use of telehealth tools in Brazil include the limited connectivity of basic health units, cultural barriers such as PHC dentist beliefs [mistrust] regarding the use of technology and case discussion with other professionals, and the low investment in the development of these services. In addition, the involvement of local managers needs to be considered, with allocation of time for telehealth activities.

Telehealth tools promote people-centered care based on the best available evidence and on the principles of quaternary prevention. The use of telehealth tools can prevent unnecessary referrals or unnecessary travel for care, in addition to improving referral information and thus accelerating the resolution of cases in which specialist consultations are in fact needed.

References

1. Nickel DA, Lima FG, Silva BB. Dental care models in Brazil. Cad Saúde Públ. 2008;24:241–6.
2. Brasil. Ministério da Saúde. Departamento de Atenção Básica. Diretrizes nacionais de saúde bucal. Brasília: Ministério da Saúde; 2004.
3. Pimentel FC, et al. Caracterização do processo de trabalho das equipes de saúde bucal em municípios de Pernambuco, Brasil, segundo porte populacional: da articulação comunitária à organização do atendimento clínico. Cad Saúde Públ. 2012;28(1):S146–57.
4. Brasil. Sistema de Informação da Atenção Básica. Portal da saúde: DATASUS. Brasília: Ministério da Saúde, 2014. Disponível em: http://datasus.saude.gov.br/sistemas-e-aplicativos/epidemiologicos/siab. Acesso em 10 maio 2016.
5. Tavares RP, et al. A organização do acesso aos serviços de saúde bucal na estratégia de saúde da família de um município da Bahia. Saúde Debate. 2013;37(99):628–35.
6. Rodrigues AAO, et al. Práticas da equipe de saúde bucal na estratégia saúde da família e a construção (des) construção da integralidade em Feira de Santana. BA Rev APS. 2010;13(4):476–85.
7. Chaves SCL, Vieira-da-Silva LM. Atenção à saúde bucal e a descentralização da saúde no Brasil: estudo de dois casos exemplares no Estado da Bahia. Cad Saúde Públ. 2007;23(5):1119–31.
8. Brasil. Ministério da Saúde. Política Nacional de Atenção Básica. Brasília: Ministério da Saúde; 2012.
9. Lorena Sobrinho JE, et al. Acesso e qualidade: avaliação das Equipes de Saúde Bucal participantes do PMAQ-AB 2012 em Pernambuco. Saúde Debate. 2015;39(104):136–46.
10. Ministério da Saúde (BR). Programa Nacional Telessaúde Brasil Redes. Custeio dos Núcleos de Telessaúde: manual instrutivo. Brasília: Ministério da Saúde; 2015.
11. Haddad AE. Experiência brasileira do Programa Nacional Telessaúde Brasil. In: Mathias I, Monteiro A, editors. Gold book [on-line]: inovação tecnológica em educação e saúde. Rio de Janeiro: UERJ; 2012.
12. Starfield B. Is US health really the best in the world? JAMA. 2000;284(4):483–5.
13. Croswell JM, et al. Cumulative incidence of false-positive results in repeated, multimodal cancer screening. Ann Fam Med. 2009;7:212–22.
14. Marcolino MS, Alkmim MB, Santos TADQ, Ribeiro AL. The telehealth network of Minas Gerais: a large-scale Brazilian public telehealth service improving access to specialised health care. Policy Focus. 2016;13(1):59–61.
15. Ministério da Saúde (BR). Portaria n. 2.546 de 27 de outubro de 2011. Redefine e amplia o Programa Telessaúde Brasil, que passa a ser denominado Programa Nacional Telessaúde Brasil Redes (Telessaúde Brasil Redes). Diário Oficial da União 2011; 28 out.
16. Wangenheim A, Barcellos CL Jr, Wagner HM, Gomes CC. Ways to implement large scale telemedicine: the Santa Catarina experience. Lat Am J Telehealth. 2009;1(3):364–77.
17. Silva NA, Santos AMG, Cortez EA, Cordeiro BC. Limites e possibilidades do ensino à distância (EaD) na educação permanente em saúde: revisão integrativa. Cienc Saúde Coletiva. 2015;20(4):1099–107.
18. Fullerton JT, Ingle HT. Evaluation strategies for midwifery education linked to digital media and distance delivery technology. J Midwifery Womens Health. 2003;48(6):426–36.
19. Schimitz CAA, D'Avila OP, Moro RG. Ferramentas de Telessaúde no Brasil.
20. Promef. Ciclo 11. Volume 4.

21. Godoy S, Mendes IAC, Hayashida M, Nogueira MS, Alves LMM. In service nursing education delivered by videoconference. J Telemed Telecare. 2004;10(5):303–5.
22. Sinclair PM, Kable A, Levette-Jones T, Booth D. The effectiveness of Internet-based e-learning on clinician behaviour and patient outcomes: a systematic review. Int J Nurs Stud. 2016;57:70–81.
23. Wong G, Greenhalgh T, Pawson R. Internet-based medical education: a realist review of what works, for whom and in what circumstances. BMC Med Educ. 2010;10(1):10–2.

Teledentistry in France: Example of the e-DENT Project

12

C. Inquimbert, E. Malthierry, G. Arzens, P. Camman, M. Charvier, F. Cuisinier, R. Delafoy, T. Dodin, V. Formont, S. Garcia, U. Gonzales, N. Huyghe, M. Lelong, B. Levallois, S. Luce, J. Pasdeloup, P.F. Perrigault, M. Pierrejean, L. Pourreyron, T. Ressouche, C. Roy, O. Roy, C. Serra, B. Tassery, H. Tassery, P. Tramini, J. Valcarcel, F. Vialla, and N. Giraudeau

C. Inquimbert
Dental Faculty, University of Montpellier, Montpellier, France
University Hospital of Montpellier, Montpellier, France
Doctoral School EDISS 205, University of Lyon 1 – Claude Bernard, Villeurbanne, France

E. Malthierry • F. Cuisinier • B. Levallois • L. Pourreyron • J. Valcarcel
Dental Faculty, University of Montpellier, Montpellier, France
University Hospital of Montpellier, Montpellier, France
Laboratory of Bioengineering and Nano-Science EA 4203, University of Montpellier, Montpellier, France

G. Arzens • S. Garcia • J. Pasdeloup • O. Roy
Dental Faculty, University of Montpellier, Montpellier, France
University Hospital of Montpellier, Montpellier, France

P. Camman • M. Charvier • R. Delafoy • T. Dodin • V. Formont • U. Gonzales
N. Huyghe • M. Lelong • M. Pierrejean • T. Ressouche • C. Roy • C. Serra
Dental Faculty, University of Montpellier, Montpellier, France

S. Luce
University Hospital of Marseille, Marseille, France

P.F. Perrigault
University Hospital of Montpellier, Montpellier, France

B. Tassery
Dental Faculty, University of Lille, Lille, France

H. Tassery
Laboratory of Bioengineering and Nano-Science EA 4203, University of Montpellier, Montpellier, France
University Hospital of Marseille, Marseille, France

N. Giraudeau (ed.), *e-Health Care in Dentistry and Oral Medicine*,
https://doi.org/10.1007/978-3-319-69450-4_12

P. Tramini
Dental Faculty, University of Montpellier, Montpellier, France
University Hospital of Montpellier, Montpellier, France
University Institute of Clinical Research, Medical Faculty (UFR),
University of Montpellier, Montpellier, France

F. Vialla
European Centre for Teaching and Research in Health Law, UMR 5815,
University of Montpellier, Montpellier, France

N. Giraudeau (✉)
Dental Faculty, University of Montpellier, Montpellier, France
University Hospital of Montpellier, Montpellier, France
Laboratory of Bioengineering and Nano-Science EA 4203,
University of Montpellier, Montpellier, France
Chaire e-Santé (e-Health), Foundation of the University of Montpellier, Montpellier, France
e-mail: nicolas.giraudeau@umontpellier.fr

Abstract

e-DENT project was born in 2012. In 2014 the first oral teleconsultation was made between a nursing home in Uzès and the University Hospital of Montpellier (60 km). Since then, more than 2000 oral teleconsultations have been realized for different kind of patients: elderly people, disabled people, inmate, patients with chronic disease, etc.

This innovative project improves the quality of oral care for several populations in the south of France. Now University Hospital of Montpellier is considered as the expert center of oral teleconsultation in France and Europe.

This chapter will resume every step of the project: legal, political, and economical aspects and all examples of populations tested in this project.

Keywords

Teledentistry • Public health • Diagnostic

12.1 Introduction

Telemedicine has been developing worldwide for several decades. Dentistry has not succeeded in keeping up with the speed of certain medical fields. However, particular trials have been conducted in different continents without ever developing into permanent practice. The Regional Health Agency (*L'Agence Régionale de Santé (ARS)*) of Languedoc-Roussillon, the University Hospital (*Centre hospitalier universitaire (CHU)*) of Montpellier and the University of Montpellier set up a project called e-DENT in an effort to organise and formalise a practice of dental telemedicine.

We outline here the important parameters in the conduct of an act of dental telemedicine. This work is the result of teamwork between several research laboratories at the University of Montpellier and the dental department of the University and Regional Hospital (*Centre hospitalier régional universitaire (CHRU)*) of Montpellier. It is based on a regional trial which enabled the execution of more than

2000 dental tele-expertise acts in 3 years. With the strength of this important stage of validation on communities with special needs (persons with loss of independence, persons with a handicap, persons with a chronic illness), dental telemedicine might be favourable for other needs: medically barren areas and communities at a distance from healthcare, for example, inmates and high-level athletes. We will discuss these possibilities in our chapter.

Telemedicine is the subject of a great number of fantasies, fears and misunderstandings. Novelty and innovation are often destabilising. However, this medical practice is not as innovative as one might think. In fact, already in the eighteenth century patients used to send letters describing their symptoms to doctors, as here the Knight of Rotalier wrote on 1 October 1771 to Dr. Tissot: 'You say that one requires much attention and skill to correctly judge the condition of a sick person when one cannot see them; your experience and your knowledge have established your reputation so well in this area that I will execute with much more confidence what you prescribe me to do than I would the orders of any other who is able to see me. I am going to describe my condition as best I possibly can' [1]. Information and communication technology used during the era was the fastest of the times: the mail service! Even if the technological side of telemedicine today was not yet current, the functioning was the same: a dispatch of information to a distant doctor in order for him to diagnose, prescribe or direct. Subsequently, each evolution of communication technology has been used for medical care: telegraph, radio and telephone. It was the inventor of this last one, Mr. Graham Bell, who solicited the first medical assistance by telephone on 10 March 1876, after having tipped sulphuric acid over himself. Only 3 years afterwards, 'the first use of the telephone in paediatric medical practice was chronicled in the Lancet journal in the form of a description of the clinical condition of a child with diphtheria' [2]. Telemedicine can be considered as a supplementary evolution of medical practice which the latter has experienced throughout the ages.

Telemedicine in dental practice is much more recent. The first trial was recorded in 1994 by the American Army [3]. It consisted of monitoring the healing of periodontal surgery. Fifteen soldiers had been sent off 120 miles away to benefit from surgery by a specialist dental surgeon. One week later, returned to their army base, the general practitioner at the base removed their stitches and took some photographic shots which were sent to the specialist at the distant location. The specialist requested only one single soldier to be sent back to him, thus avoiding at the same time the cost and time lost for the other 14 soldiers. A certain number of trials have been conducted worldwide since this date [4] and notably in France [5, 6]. Dental telemedicine has seen considerable development in the past months, and we take advantage of the involvement in this work to outline and explain the trial that we have been conducting in Languedoc-Roussillon for several years now (first teleconsultation on 28 April 2014).

To this end, we will return to the dental telemedicine trial undertaken in the Languedoc-Roussillon region being piloted by the public health department of the Centre for Dental Treatment, Teaching and Research (*Centre de Soins d'Enseignement et de Recherche Dentaire (CSERD)*) of the University and Regional Hospital of Montpellier.

We will successively outline the legal framework, the technological and technical system used and its functioning and the current economic model of telemedicine in France, concluding by returning briefly to the different trials conducted.

12.2 Telemedicine, a Fundamental Legal Tool for Healthcare Democracy

12.2.1 A Clear Legal Framework

Telemedicine has been clearly defined legally since the *HPST* Act (Act of 21 July 2009 reforming Hospitals and Patient, Health and Regional Affairs) and the creation of Article L.6316-1 of the Public Health Code (*Code de la Santé Publique (CSP)*). Here the legislator revisits the previously applied article (Act of 13 August 2004 concerning health insurance) to improve the definition of telemedicine, but most importantly, this article was followed by a decree of application dated 19 October 2010 (Decree n° 2010-1229). It is the publication of this decree which will allow for the development of telemedicine on national territory. In fact, this decree tables the different telemedicine consultations and their organisation and sets the stage for possible financing of this new type of medical activity.

'Telemedicine is a distance medical practice using information and communication technology', as set out in Article L.6316-1 of the Public Health Code. Just as all medical activities, it must adhere to regional health policy. The Regional Health Agency is the guarantor of this strategic and policy thinking. The development of telemedicine activities must therefore be in line with the objectives of the Regional Health Project (*Projet Régional de Santé (PRS)*) and in particular with the Regional Telemedicine Programme (*Programme Régional de Télémédecine (PRT)*) which organises the implementation of the different distance medical practices. A telemedicine contract must be drafted for each telemedicine activity and frame the practice, organise the activities and connect the different parties.

Five telemedicine acts are defined in the first article of the telemedicine decree (Art. R.6316-1 of the Public Health Code). They consist of teleconsultation, tele-expertise, medical tele-surveillance, medical tele-aid and emergency medical response. We will only define here the first two acts.

Teleconsultation is a medical act which allows a medical professional to perform a consultation for a patient at a distance. The latter can be accompanied by a healthcare professional. Teleconsultations must necessarily be performed in a synchronous mode. This specification was only added in 2016 by the Ministry of Health in order to make a teleconsultation as close to a 'classical' consultation as possible.

Tele-expertise is an exchange of medical information between medical professionals with the aim of improving patient care. One must differentiate between tele-expertise and a medical staff meeting by videoconference. Tele-expertise acts can be carried out directly or asynchronously.

For the sake of organisational simplicity and cost, we have chosen to carry out asynchronous tele-expertise acts.

12.2.2 The Parties

As tabled by Article L.6316-1 of the Public Health Code, a medical professional must be present. These professionals are referred to in the Public Health Code, in the first book of Part Four. Here we find doctors, dental surgeons and midwives. By their sides, healthcare professionals can participate in a telemedicine activity. These professionals are referred to in the Public Health Code in the third book also of Part Four. We find here National Qualified Nurses (*Infirmiers Diplômés d'Etat (IDE)*), carers and a certain number of other professions. It is important to note that, until the Health Act of 2016, no healthcare profession was directly associated with dental healthcare. This new health law amended this peculiarity since dental assistants have at last been included in the Public Health Code. On the other hand, our country has not yet had the opportunity of benefitting from the expertise of dental hygienists, contrary to nearly all 'industrialised' countries.

Dental surgeons have therefore the legal capacity to participate in a telemedicine activity. At their side, *IDE*s appear to be the professionals of choice. In fact, in their own role, they have the capacity to undertake 'oral care with application of non-medicinal products' (Art. R.4311-5 28° of the Public Health Code) and, in the framework of a protocol or an order, to undertake 'oral care with application of medicinal products and, where necessary, instrumental aids' (Art. R.4311-7 25° of the Public Health Code). The legislator therefore permits *IDE*s to do a certain number of tasks within oral healthcare. We also note that an *IDE* can 'contribute to the gathering of useful information from other professionals, and particularly from doctors for their diagnosis and an evaluation of the effects of their prescriptions' (Art. R.4311-2 2° of the Public Health Code). The recording of videos of a patient's oral cavity is therefore part of the 'legal' capacities of an *IDE*.

This precise legal framing of telemedicine is particular to France. Other countries have not yet legislated precisely on the practice of telemedicine. Some American states have put a framework in place but nothing at the federal level. This does not prevent practices from developing but causes a certain confusion in the definition of dental telemedicine or 'tele-dentistry'. Out of concern for precision, we define dental telemedicine as a clinical practice of dentistry at a distance. We are therefore excluding from this definition preventative activities carried out with the aid of digital application or even blogs or other specialised websites that we could class in the category of oral e-Health. Furthermore, dental telemedicine does not include distance learning aimed at dental surgeons, as part of their initial or ongoing training, that we would class in the category of e-learning and which is not really a clinical dental practice.

12.2.3 The Main Observed Principles of Health Law

With telemedicine being considered by the legislator as a fully fledged medical practice, it is crucial that the healthcare professionals involved in this type of activity respect confidentiality, clearly inform patients and procure their consent when performing a medical check by telemedicine and when using information and communication technology for transferring or saving this personal medical data.

12.3 The System

12.3.1 Inclusion of a Technological Third Party

12.3.1.1 An Equipped Healthcare Professional

As we have just indicated, it is necessary to have an *IDE* at the patient's side in order to record the information which will enable the dental surgeon's diagnosis. It is obvious that in order to make a quality diagnosis at a distance, the practitioner needs good visibility of the oral cavity and teeth of the patient. For that, we decided to use an intra-oral camera using a fluorescent light (Soprocare®). This camera makes caries lesions visible, even precursory ones [7, 8], as well as gingival inflammations and dental plaque. This element is vital to making a diagnosis from a distance.

12.3.1.2 Specific Equipment

A clinical study was conducted in order to validate remote diagnosis with the aid of an intra-oral camera using fluorescence [9]. One hundred patients from the Centre for Dental Treatment, Teaching and Research at the University and Regional Hospital of Montpellier had a 'classical' consultation with a dental surgeon making a precise report of caries lesions using the ICDAS classification (www.icdas.org), and then a sixth-year student took videos of each sector of the patient's mouth so that another practitioner could analyse the videos remotely. This study showed a specificity of 79%, a sensitivity of 99% with a negative predictive value of 94% and a positive predictive value of 95%. This study is being carried out under the same conditions in Japan at the Kyushu University.

12.3.1.3 Necessary Technical Organisation

In addition to this intra-oral camera, a specific dentistry specialised telemedicine platform is required to facilitate the recording of patient data and videos. This platform also enables ensuring the security of the transfer and saving of data as the telemedicine decree stipulates. For our trial, we worked with e-DENT® software from the company e-DENTECH (Montpellier, France).

12.3.2 Functioning

12.3.2.1 An Asynchronous Act

The workflow of a dental tele-expertise act is similar to a tele-expertise act in another specialty. A requesting professional is at the patient's side in order to facilitate the recording of information necessary for the diagnosis, and a requested professional is at a distant location and will perform the medical act of dental diagnosis. The particularity that we find with this specialty is the asynchrony of the tele-expertise act. In fact, there is no medical necessity for the requested professional to be connected at the same time as the requesting professional and the patient. There is no vital urgency in dentistry, and the asynchronous performance of the tele-expertise act allows for greater flexibility in its organisation. First of all, in the human time required, the *IDE* can take the time needed to collect the information and, in particular, the recording of videos which sometimes takes longer especially for dependent patients. Moreover, in the case of asynchrony, requested professionals are not waiting in front of their screen and are therefore able to optimise their time and make analyses of the teleconsultations according to their schedule. Subsequently, the establishments in which the tele-expertise acts are recorded do not require a Wi-Fi connection. This functioning therefore allows a greater freedom regarding the place where the recording of videos is performed (residents' bedrooms, dedicated room, etc.). Finally, carrying out a telemedicine act in direct mode requires a secure internet connection with very good quality. This fact makes the cost of connection rise quite considerably.

12.3.2.2 A Formalised Workflow

More specifically, once the oral clean-up has been performed, the *IDE*, previously trained in the main principles of dentistry, in the use of software and in handling an intra-oral camera, records the required information. This stage is facilitated by the protocol established in the software. The following are requested:

- Information concerning the patient's identity. The remote dental surgeon must know the identity of the patient he is taking responsibility for, as in classical practice. Furthermore, the patient also knows which professional is going to perform his examination. Freedom of choice of practitioner must always be respected.
- Information on patient's general condition: chronic diseases, allergies, medication, possible malnourishment.
- Information on patient's cognitive state.
- Information on patient's dental history and oral hygiene: wearing of removable dentures, frequency of brushing, pain, tooth mobility.
- Compilation of the odontogram (dental chart). It is important to be sure that if a tooth is not visible on the video, it is because the tooth is not in the mouth and not because the requesting professional did not film it.
- Recording a video by sector, at the least, using the camera's different modes of fluorescence. Other videos or photos can be included if necessary.

Once the visit has been undertaken and the secure Wi-Fi or line connection established, the data is transmitted to an *ASIP Santé*[1]-approved secure central server.

[1] National French digital health agency.

The requested dental surgeon connects with a username and password to make sure that the videos are analysed by the practitioner the patients chose to perform their tele-expertise diagnosis. As a strong authentication from the requested professional is required by the legislator, a certificate of authentication was therefore added to the computer which allows the 'tele-dentist' to connect. This method was preferred rather than the use of the healthcare professional card since it does not require a reader and medical professionals do not always have their card with them, particularly hospital practitioners.

12.3.2.3 The Starting Point for an Adapted Dental Treatment Plan

The specialist can now perform the act of tele-expertise. The analysis of videos and different information gathered by the *IDE* will allow him to make a diagnosis and recommend a treatment plan. This may include a dental treatment according to the dental and general pathology of the patient as well as a recommended care plan adapted to the patient. In fact, depending on the cognitive state and general condition of the patient and accounting for the patient's acceptance of the camera, it is very useful to be able to orient the patient directly towards the most suitable treatment type: private practice, private practice using nitrous oxide, deep sedation or general anaesthetic. The scheduling and prioritisation of the treatment are proposed. All this information is then collated in an automatically generated report and sent to the patient's file. If an appointment with a dental surgeon is prescribed, the patient is free to choose the practitioner who will perform the treatment. In the case of medico-welfare establishments, the protocols for booking specialist appointments are well organised, and the tele-expertise plays the role of trigger.

12.4 Building a Permanent Economic Model

The growth in dental telemedicine raises the question of creating a permanent economic model, which entails cost and revenue redistribution in this new process [10]. The current economic model is actually based on non-permanent financing, in the context of the support of the pilot trial by the Regional Health Agencies. Firstly, to ensure sustainable development of this new medical practice, consideration must be given to the redistribution of revenue between the parties, for clinicians in particular, and to the inclusion of the acts of the *IDE* recording essential information for the diagnosis by the dentist. Next, new costs need to be taken into account resulting from the arrival of two new entrants in the process: the software publisher and the data host. The recognition of telemedicine acts and their financing in the context of pricing per act are crucial questions. It is therefore necessary to distinguish the challenges concerning the financing of technological platforms required for setting up dental telemedicine from the question of the pricing of these acts and their financing [11].

Thus far, the Ministry of Health has proposed a remuneration for tele-expertise acts: a flat fee of €40 per patient per year. This fee is to be shared between the *IDE*s who will gather the information and the remote dental surgeon who will perform the medical act. At each tele-expertise act, the *IDE* will receive €1, and the dental surgeon will receive the remainder of the €40 at year end. For example, if Mr. John Smith receives benefits from two tele-expertise acts in 2018, the *IDE* who recorded the information will receive €2 at year end and the dentist €38. Note that a classical dental consultation is priced by medical insurance at €23.

It is important to underline that a tele-expertise act takes between 5 and 15 min for the practitioner.

12.5 Trial Setup in Languedoc-Roussillon

In order to assess the technical and clinical feasibility as well as the acceptability and the organisation of such an activity [12], the Regional Health Agency of Languedoc-Roussillon set up a trial on a regional scale. This was carried out by the Centre for Dental Treatment, Teaching and Research at the University and Regional Hospital of Montpellier with the participation of the Cooperative Health Group e-Health (*Groupement de Coopération Sanitaire (GCS) e-Santé*), different research laboratories at the University of Montpellier (*LBN, CEERDS, MRM*) and the Regional Health Professionals Union of Dental Surgeons (*Union Régionale des Professionnels de Santé des Chirurgiens-Dentistes*) of Languedoc-Roussillon. It was anticipated that the residents of the eight Aged Care Nursing Homes (*Etablissements Hébergeant des Personnes Agées Dépendantes (EHPAD)*) managed by the Hospital Centre of Uzès, four Aged Care Nursing Homes managed by the Hospital Centre of the Bassin de Thau and three Specialist Care Homes in the Department of Aude might benefit from two tele-expertise appointments 6 months apart in order to see whether dental hygiene had improved and if the prescribed care had been followed. As well, it was also requested that 100 detainees from the Villeneuve-lès-Maguelone detention centre be provided the benefit of this tele-expertise experience at the time of the initial medical visit upon arrival in incarceration. For this, financing was assumed by the Regional Health Agency in order to take responsibility for the expenses relating to equipment, coordination and the nurse time required for the data collection.

During this trial between January 2014 and November 2015, more than 750 persons were able to benefit from a tele-expertise procedure.

12.5.1 Benefit for Persons with Special Needs

Amongst the aged, we have been able to ascertain a real acceptance of participating in these tele-expertise procedures. They appreciate the fact of not having to travel for a dental check-up but mostly because it is a person with whom they have daily contact who collects the information and records the videos thanks to the intra-oral camera. Indeed, in the chosen institutions, a nurse was trained to perform the recordings. We also find this same situation in the institutions for handicapped persons and particularly for intellectually disabled persons.

12.5.2 Benefit for Inmates

For persons detained by the law, tele-expertise procedures were above all beneficial in the organisation of the prison health service. Despite the regulatory obligation to perform dental check-ups of all prisoners arriving in detention [13], this examination was not practised at the detention centre of Villeneuve-lès-Maguelone mainly due to lack of time for the dental surgeon.

With the setup of tele-expertise procedures in July 2014, all detainees were able to benefit from a dental check-up. This enabled prioritisation of the treatments to be carried out. As well, this resulted in a reduction in the number of dental emergencies and consequently alleviated the dentist's scheduling which allowed him to improve his treatment sessions.

Alongside the Regional Health Agency trial, we tested tele-expertise procedures on other communities:

- 100 patients from the day ward of the psychiatric centre at the University Hospital of Montpellier
- 23 patients waiting to have a heart valve fitted in the cardiology centre at the University Hospital of Montpellier
- 50 patients from the treatment centre for drug addiction at the University Hospital of Montpellier
- 65 patients from the centre for eating disorders at the University Hospital of Montpellier
- 350 male and female players from the National French Basketball teams

12.5.3 Benefit for the Chronically Ill

In these various centres, we were able to confirm that dental tele-expertise procedures allow for an ideal starting point for the organisation of a dental care plan. These patients suffering from a general medical condition often have difficulty finding a practitioner who will take care of them in a private practice because of the difficulty with treatment, either from a technical or psychological aspect. Thanks to the tele-expertise procedures carried out in these centres, we were able to more easily motivate patients to seek treatment but also to simplify their care in the university hospital's dental centre when their situation required it. In fact, since we know the dental condition of the patient as well as his general condition, we can more easily organise his visit to the centre and prescribe the necessary prophylactic antibiotics, if required, so as to reduce the number of appointments whilst increasing their efficiency.

12.5.4 Benefit for High-Level Athletes

As part of a project in partnership with the French Basketball Federation (*Fédération Française de Basketball*), we carried out tele-expertise procedures with the cohort of male and female players in the National French Basketball teams from the U19s to the A teams.

The request from the federal doctor was to be able to make an early diagnosis of dental problems in order to avoid pain when travelling abroad and to reduce the risk of player downtime due to dental pain as has been the case in the past.

The community of high-level athletes is one with a high risk of dental problems mainly because of their heavy consumption of sugary drinks, their habit of snacking and reduced salivation during exertion [14]. Moreover, it seems that their very busy schedule due to their numerous training sessions makes a visit to the dentist difficult. Even if the benefit was not the same amongst these athletes as within the aforementioned communities, it is clear from this trial that the players particularly appreciated being able to simplify their access to dental consultation. The gathering of information is done in the treatment room and the results given back to them at their monthly appointment with the doctor (except in the case of a dental emergency).

12.5.5 Next Communities to Be Targeted

Other trials should see the light of day in the next months on children in the schools of Montpellier, agricultural workers and soldiers.

Conclusion

Dental telemedicine, and in particular tele-expertise, is an innovative public health tool which must be integrated into the care of a certain number of special communities. It is now important that the profession of dental surgeons, their representatives, their unions and learned societies assume ownership of this tool and ensure it is well used. One must follow the example of doctors who have drafted white books or recommendations about good practices in telemedicine use. Mistakes and difficulties encountered by doctors must serve dentists in speeding up the creation of an organisational and clinical framework for the practice of dental telemedicine.

Now that the clinical, organisational and legal validations have been made by this trial, it is important to continue to use telemedicine in different public health situations in order to know its limits.

References

1. Bibliothèque Cantonale Universitaire de Lausanne (BCUL). Département des manuscrits, Fonds Tissot.
2. HAS. Prescription médicamenteuse par téléphone (ou téléprescription) dans le cadre de la régulation médicale. Haute Autorité de Santé; 2009 févr, p. 23.
3. Alipour-Rocca L, Kudryk V, Morris T. TME3/347: a teledentistry consultation system and continuing dental education via Internet. J Med Internet Res [Internet]. 1999 [cité 6 févr 2013];1(1). Disponible sur: http://www.ncbi.nlm.nih.gov/pmc/articles/PMC1761814/.
4. Glassman P. Virtual dental home. J Californian Dent Assoc. 2012;40(7):565–6.

5. Giraudeau N, Valcarcel J, Tassery H, Levallois B, Cuisinier F, Tramini P, et al. Projet e-DENT: téléconsultation bucco-dentaire en EHPAD. Eur Res Telemed Rech Eur En Télémédecine. 2014;3(2):51–6.
6. Le populaire. Le programme européen LivInWell a dressé un premier bilan d'étape au CMN de Sainte-Feyre [Internet]. 2015 [cité 20 oct 2015]. Disponible sur: http://www.lepopulaire.fr/limousin/actualite/departement/creuse/gueret/2015/06/26/le-programme-europeen-livinwell-a-dresse-un-premier-bilan-detape-au-cmn-de-sainte-feyre-hier_11497672.html.
7. Rechmann P, Charland D, Rechmann BMT, Featherstone JDB. Performance of laser fluorescence devices and visual examination for the detection of occlusal caries in permanent molars. J Biomed Opt. 2012;17(3):0360061–5.
8. Panayotov I, Terrer E, Salehi H, Tassery H, Yachouh J, Cuisinier FJG, et al. In vitro investigation of fluorescence of carious dentin observed with a Soprolife® camera. Clin Oral Investig. 2013;17(3):757–63. https://doi.org/10.1007/s00784-012-0770-9. Epub 2012 Aug 2.
9. Roy C, Giraudeau N, Pourreyron L, Perrigault P-F, Tassery H, Cuisinier F, et al. Etude clinique comparative entre une consultation classique et une téléconsultation. Alpha Oméga News; 2016.
10. Chen S, Cheng A, Mehta K. A review of telemedicine business models. Telemed E-Health. 2013;19(4):287–97.
11. Horquin T. Les conditions d'émergence des marchés de la télémédecine: entre territoires de santé, projets d'expérimentation et écosystèmes d'affaires. Telecom Paris Tech; 2011.
12. Ologeanu-Taddei R, Bourdon I, Kimble C, Giraudeau N. The acceptability of teleconsultation in teledentistry: a case study. In: Cruz-Cunha M, Miranda I, editors. Encyclopedia of e-health and telemedicine. Hershey: IGI Global; 2015.
13. Ministère de la santé et des sports, Ministère de la justice et des libertés. Plan d'actions strategiques 2010-2014: politique de santé pour les personnes placées sous main de justice [Internet]. Ministère de la santé et des sports; 2010 [cité 26 févr 2013]. p. 84. Disponible sur: http://www.sante.gouv.fr/IMG/pdf/Plan_actions_strategiques_detenus.pdf.
14. Haute Autorité de Santé. Stratégies de prévention de la carie dentaire. Haute Autorité de Santé; 2010.

Printed by Printforce, the Netherlands